Praise for *Keep*

"An amazing and positively effective book. It will change the way you think about the weight you have carried around or want to lose."
—George J. Pratt, Ph.D., coauthor of *Instant Emotional Healing*,
    and Chairman, Psychology, Scripps Memorial Hospital

"A clearly written guide enabling overweight people to draw upon internal resources for accomplishing and maintaining weight loss . . . A major addition to the self-help literature."
    —Vincent J. Felitti, M.D., California Institutes of
        Preventive Medicines

"I found this to be the best written book on mind/body approaches applied to weight management ever written."
—Arnold Singer, M.D., Internal Medicine, Kaiser Permanente

"It's hard to imagine someone following the book's plan and NOT succeeding . . . It's so refreshing to find a book on weight loss that gives the reader a step-by-step way to deal with the deeper issues that created the weight problem."
    —Susan Horowitz, M.D., Children's Hospital San Diego

Brian Alman holds a Ph.D. in clinical psychology and has been in private practice for twenty-five years. His previous books, *Thin Meditations*, *Six Steps to Freedom*, *Self-Hypnosis*, and *A Clinical Hypnosis Primer*, have sold more than 250,000 copies. He is affiliated with the Kaiser Permanente health-care organization, whose Positive Choice weight-loss program will be featured in Dr. Alman's forthcoming infomercial. He lives in San Diego, California.

Stephen Montgomery is a Ph.D. in literature, an award-winning English teacher, and a National Endowment for the Humanities fellow. He is the editor of the bestseller *Please Understand Me*, and the author of *The Pygmalion Project* and *People Patterns*.

"Dr. Alman does not offer 'band aid' solutions to sustained weight loss. Rather, he addresses fundamental and thus 'root issues' underlying the inability to keep it off."
—Wayne Beach, Ph.D., San Diego University

"Everyone looking to lose weight and improve their state of well-being without toxic drugs, surgical distortion of digestion, or untoward manipulation of nutrition would benefit from the learnings within *Keep It Off*."
—Bob Hogan, M.D., Kaiser Permanente

"This book is an essential tool for people who are serious, not just for weight loss, but about changing any negative or compulsive pattern. I highly recommend it."
—Dr. Peter Lambrou, Ph.D., Scripps Memorial Hospital

Also by Brian Alman

Thin Meditations
Six Steps to Freedom
Self-Hypnosis
A Clinical Hypnosis Primer

KEEP IT OFF

Your Key
to
Weight Loss for Life

BRIAN ALMAN, Ph.D.
WITH STEPHEN MONTGOMERY, Ph.D.

A PLUME BOOK

PLUME
Published by Penguin Group
Penguin Group (USA) Inc., 375 Hudson Street, New York, New York 10014, U.S.A.
Penguin Group (Canada), 10 Alcorn Avenue, Toronto, Canada M4V 3B2
(a division of Pearson Penguin Canada Inc.)
Penguin Books Ltd, 80 Strand, London WC2R 0RL, England
Penguin Group (Australia), 250 Camberwell Road, Camberwell,
Penguin Ireland, 25 St Stephen's Green, Dublin 2, Ireland (a division of Penguin Books Ltd)
Victoria 3124, Australia (a division of Pearson Australia Group Pty Ltd)
Penguin Books India Pvt Ltd, 11 Community Centre,
Panchsheel Park, New Delhi – 110 017, India
Penguin Books (NZ), Cnr Airborne and Rosedale Roads, Albany,
Auckland 1310, New Zealand (a division of Pearson New Zealand Ltd)
Penguin Books (South Africa) (Pty) Ltd, 24 Sturdee Avenue,
Rosebank, Johannesburg 2196, South Africa

Penguin Books Ltd, Registered Offices: 80 Strand, London WC2R 0RL, England

Published by Plume, a member of Penguin Group (USA) Inc.
Previously published in a Dutton edition.

First Plume Printing, January 2005
1 3 5 7 9 10 8 6 4 2

Copyright © Brian Alman, 2004
All rights reserved

℗ REGISTERED TRADEMARK—MARCA REGISTRADA

CIP data is available.
ISBN 0-525-94812-0 (hc.)
ISBN 0-452-28633-6 (pbk.)

Printed in the United States of America
Original hardcover design by Leonard Telesca

PUBLISHER'S NOTE
Neither the publisher nor the author is engaged in rendering professional advice or services to the individual reader. The ideas, procedures, and suggestions contained in this book are not intended as a substitute for consulting with your physician. All matters regarding your health require medical supervision. Neither the author nor the publisher shall be liable or responsible for any loss or damage allegedly arising from any information or suggestion in this book.

Contents

Acknowledgments

Keep It Off is the culmination of twenty-five years of helping people lose weight and keep it off. I continue to be 100% committed to helping people help themselves as it relates to living well, learning new things, and resolving the challenges of losing weight and keeping it off. It has been the central focus of all my work with mind/body approaches, relaxation, visualization, guided imagery, and self-hypnosis. I have been very fortunate to work with the most comprehensive weight-loss program in the United States, Kaiser Permanente's Positive Choice Wellness Center, and specifically with the two people that started it all: Vincent Felitti, M.D. (father of the ACE study on obesity), and Kathy Jakstis (creative director and organizational wizard).

Thanks to my wife, Tracie, for always living and sharing your heartfelt style in such a positive and accepting way. You integrate your positive lifestyle so naturally; focusing on what's right about people, with your openness to your imagination and new ideas, and caring deeply about your relationships. You inspire me and many others to keep things in perspective by seeing what is practical and at the same time seeing what is possible.

• • •

Thank you to my small-sized, medium-sized, and grown-up–sized kids, who continually inspire me while keeping me humble: Alaina Rose, Deanna, Brittany, Mike, Shishana, and Rebecca.

Thanks to Steve Montgomery, Ph.D., for the extraordinary writing skill and wise counsel on the content of this book. Steve is a wonderful writer, has a thorough understanding of what it takes to help people help themselves, and has written extensively on the importance of individual styles of change. I know he was assisted on many occasions by his soul partner and wife, Jan. Thanks to both of you for dedicating your time and energy to helping make *Keep It Off* the book that it is.

Thanks to Bill Gladstone, literary agent and friend, and his entire staff at Waterside Productions in Cardiff-by-the-Sea, California. Bill's focus and determination made sure we had the best weight-loss book possible. Bill's understanding that other weight-loss books have failed in helping people keep the weight off allowed him to support my vision with strength and direction.

Special thanks to Reno Rolle, who continually inspires me with his integrity and has moved the informercial, marketing, and availability of *Keep It Off* to people who want the ultimate key to losing weight (inside and out).

Thanks to Brian Tart and Julie Doughty from Penguin Group USA in New York. Their expertise and patience helped keep this project on course and the sailing smooth.

Thanks to my colleagues, clients, students, and teachers, particularly Dr. Milton H. Erickson, who took me into his home and helped me grow into a teacher of self-hypnosis and a man.

And thanks to all the people who will read this book and keep it off. . . .

Introduction:
The Missing Ingredient

... we are a package of thinking and feelings housed within this body that is called you and me. In order to make any change for the better, all of the parts of ourselves must be addressed for that change to become permanent.

—Deepak Chopra

What's the first thing that comes to mind when you think of losing weight? Is it counting calories? Diet centers? Diet pills and plans? Starting an exercise program for the twentieth time (with that new machine you bought for Christmas)? You've probably tried some or all of these methods—and many others—with little or only temporary success.

Actually, many diet and exercise programs work pretty well. The real problem is not the ineffectiveness of the program, but the dieter's *inability to stay with the program* once the weight has been lost. The rate of relapse is disturbingly high—right around 95 percent according to the weight-loss industry's own figures.

Why do we begin overeating in the first place? And why, even if we lose the weight, is it so hard to keep it off? What's the missing ingredient that keeps all these weight-loss plans and programs from making a real, lasting difference?

To help answer these questions, let me introduce you to a client of mine, Mary.

The Case of Mary

Mary wasn't at all happy with her weight, and she was looking for help. When we first talked in my office, she told me that four years ago, when she was thirty-five, she weighed a comfortable, attractive 125 pounds. Then she explained how she began gradually putting on weight, until she weighed over 170 pounds.

And she didn't know what to do about it.

She had tried all the popular diets, diet books, diet programs, and diet centers, and nothing had worked for more than a few months. She would lose weight, gain it all back and more, lose weight again, then gain back more, and on and on, caught in a vicious cycle of "yo-yo" dieting. Plus, she was becoming obsessed with losing weight—with food, fat, calories—and she was ending up with nothing but feelings of failure for her efforts.

How could such an intelligent person, and one seemingly in control in other areas of her life, get so stuck in a rut? As Mary took a deep breath, closed her eyes, and told me more of her story, she started getting to the bottom of things.

Mary's Story—"More Sad Than Happy"

Mary was successful and satisfied with her job, but a difficult divorce four years earlier, child custody battles, and a stressful remarriage had left her feeling, as she said, "more sad than happy lately."

And she soon realized that there were other emotions weighing her down. Raised a Catholic, she felt guilty about being divorced; she was still angry at her ex-husband for what she felt were injustices; and she was exhausted and sometimes over-whelmed trying to raise her daughters and keep a career going. She acknowledged, probably for the first time, how empty she felt in her life. And she also admitted that her weight gain had not been gradual (as she first told me), but had occurred in a few short months, right after her separation four years ago.

Why, then, had Mary gained weight? Why had she put the weight on when she did, and why couldn't she keep it off?

The Answers Are Always Inside

The answer is that, in those difficult years, overeating made Mary feel better about her life, if only for a short while.

It was her way of distracting herself from her troubles, her way of stuffing down her unwanted feelings, her way of expressing her biting anger at her selfish ex-husband, her way of quieting her negative thinking (even though it was only temporary), her way of filling up the emptiness she felt in her personal life, her way of feeling less lonely at night.

In short, overeating became Mary's most effective way of dealing with her problems, given her coping skills at the time. Considering all the troubles she was faced with, and consider-ing she didn't know of any better way to handle them, I would say that Mary was wise and resourceful, and did a great job of caring for herself and helping herself through this tough period of her life.

Is There a Part of You Like Mary?

Mary's is a familiar story, and it can help us all understand that, in most cases, gaining weight is not the problem, but the solution to our problems.

Overeating, or eating unhealthy foods, is not usually caused by physical appetite. It's caused by emotional need. For Mary, as for millions (estimated at 70 percent of American adults and 30 percent of American kids), overeating is a coping mechanism, a practical and positive way we have of dealing with the many stresses in our personal, family, and social lives.

Associating food with comfort and protection is a normal response learned in childhood, probably at the breast or the bottle. And so when faced with life's difficulties we often turn to food for help, or as a simple form of self-treatment. We even call our portions "helpings," "treats," and we say "help yourself" at the table. In a sense, all food is "comfort" food.

Unfortunately, by comforting or treating ourselves with food, we ignore meaningful signals we're trying to send to ourselves— our real call for help—that we need to get to the root of the problem.

Shedding the Emotional Weight

It has become clear from my work at Kaiser Permanente's Wellness Center in San Diego, California, that the root cause of overeating is almost always repressed feelings. Your body is the natural receptacle for repressed, suppressed, or unresolved feelings, and carrying around this kind of emotional weight often creates a need, an emotional hunger, that puts on physical weight as well.

In other words, when you're miserable inside, when shame and guilt and fear and resentment (and more) are silently "eating" at you, you try to make yourself feel better by indulging yourself with food. And the more feelings you've trapped inside, and the longer you've suffered with them, the more you want and need to eat.

This explains why the diet plan relapse rate is so high. All the popular plans will help you lose unwanted pounds—for a little while—but unless you deal with your repressed feelings, unless you do something to lighten the emotional weight you're carrying inside, you'll go right back to soothing and satisfying yourself with food.

So this is it—the missing ingredient that goes unrecognized and thus unaddressed in all other weight-loss programs. To make any lasting change in your body weight, you need to dig into your buried feelings and discover what they are, what part they've played in your life, and how they've brought you to where you are now. Only when you're willing to face and to resolve your emotional issues, to finish the unfinished business in your life—people, hurts, mistakes, wrongs, and so on—will you be able to get free of your old eating habits and keep the weight off.

The formula is simple but powerful: If you'll allow yourself to shed your old emotional and psychological baggage, the physical weight will naturally follow. If you want to lose weight and keep it off, to win the battle once and for all, you need to start at the beginning, with the emotional healing that must take place before you can start to eat, exercise, and care for yourself healthily. If you'll look deeply into the underlying emotional causes of your overeating, you can actually turn your weight problem into a doorway, or a bridge, to becoming healthier and happier—permanently.

What's the Secret?

The secret to losing weight and keeping it off is quite simply to start respecting yourself, caring for yourself, even loving yourself, without conditions, restrictions, or requirements. Once you start to love yourself truly as you are, with all your strengths and weaknesses—pounds and all—you'll naturally start to take better care of yourself, mind and body, heart and soul. And you'll find yourself feeling healthy, happy, peaceful, positive, light, calm, and energetic. It's nothing short of miraculous.

But the miracle of unconditional self-love can be almost impossible to achieve for most of us, weighed down as we are with a lifetime of stifled feelings, negative messages, and self-criticism. So to start you on the road to self-love, self-care, and permanent weight loss, I've devised the Keep It Off Weight-Loss Program, a four-phase plan that uses the power of self-hypnosis to help you access your inner resources to make these amazing and lasting changes in your life.

Step by step, you'll learn to:

1. Become **Aware** of your body, mind, feelings, and true self. Become relaxed and honest about your relationship with food; begin listening to the inner signals you've been ignoring or avoiding for years; recognize the emotional issues that are sabotaging your happiness and self-confidence; and discover how to stop your past from controlling your present.

2. Begin to **Accept** yourself (and your body) as you are, a vital step in freeing yourself from the triggers of overeating, and in coming to understand, and to embrace, the true, authentic you. Begin connecting with your inner wisdom; stop judging yourself with critical thoughts and feelings; and discover how to turn negative thinking into positive thinking.

3. Let yourself **Express** your true self safely, simply, comfortably, easily, and positively. Start releasing your pent-up thoughts and feelings; give a voice to all the conflicting messages in your head; let go of some conscious control to gain a natural freedom and balance; and discover yourself feeling alive and rejuvenated in the present.

4. Find ways to **Resolve** your unfinished personal issues once and for all, and learn how to carry these new tools and techniques with you forever. Reorganize the way you interact with yourself and others; and discover how to use the stresses swirling through your life to help you develop more positive and creative eating habits.

My experience with helping thousands of overweight people, both in my private practice and at Kaiser Permanente, has proven to me that the learning you will experience in the Keep It Off Weight-Loss Program is genuine, lasting, and can result in inner and outer transformation—something often dreamed about, but seldom realized.

Be Prepared

A word of warning: Prepare yourself for something entirely new and remarkably effective. Unlike all the diet pills, plans, and products you've heard of, or maybe tried, the Keep It Off Weight-Loss Program will show you how to find *within yourself* the power to lose weight and keep it off. It will give you the tools you need to open some new doors in your life, perhaps to reopen some old ones, all to open your heart, mind, body, and soul to positive changes.

Part I of this book will teach you the fundamentals of self-hypnosis, because self-hypnosis is the best way to open the lines of communication with your inner emotional world. Read the eight short chapters in Part I completely and give yourself time to digest and practice the methods and techniques they describe.

Once you've learned the basics of self-hypnosis, you'll have all the skills you need to make the most of my Keep It Off Weight-Loss Program presented in Part II.

Being seriously overweight is a nightmare for so many of us. But the good news is that, with the help of self-hypnosis, you have the ability to solve your weight problems safely, effectively, and permanently. The natural instinct for health and happiness you were born with is waiting to be freed and empowered.

Mary's New Life

As for Mary, she has lost her unwanted weight and has succeeded in keeping it off for over a year. By working with self-hypnosis through the four essential phases of self-change—heightened Awareness, unconditional Acceptance, free Expression, and creative Resolution—Mary took the very issues that had driven her to overeat and used them to build a bridge to new feelings, ideas, behaviors, opportunities, and answers. She learned how to stop the vicious cycle of yo-yo dieting, how to transcend her "stuck" places, and how to move on with self-love and self-confidence. She took what I like to call a breath of "fresh **AAER**" and learned how to lose weight and keep it off.

Mary is a real person, one of the many I've worked with at Kaiser Permanente, and here is what she wrote me recently:

Dear Dr. Alman,

I just wanted to thank you on my birthday. What I have learned from you during this last year makes me feel like this is my first birthday of a happy life that can continue for the rest of my life!

Thank you so much!

Mary

KEEP IT OFF

PART I

Learning Self-Hypnosis

The patient's primary task is to develop their unconscious potential. Everyone is an individual in the process of development. Hypnosis is an experience in which people receive something from themselves.

—Milton H. Erickson

CHAPTER 1

What Is Self-Hypnosis?

Welcome to the start of a journey to permanent weight loss using the power of self-hypnosis.

If you're investigating self-hypnosis for the first time, you should know that you're about to learn how to make dramatic and positive changes in your life. In the matter of a few weeks working with self-hypnosis, you're going to discover how to take care of yourself, how to break old habits and learn new ones, and how to feel the joy again of being you.

And in the process of becoming healthier and happier, you're going to learn the secret—missing in *all* diet programs—of how to lose weight and keep it off for good.

This might sound like a miracle, and yet self-hypnosis is not magical, is not mysterious, is in no way occult. It's actually a common skill that anyone can master quite easily. It's no more difficult than riding a bicycle, something almost all of us learned to do as children. We might have been a bit unsteady and uncertain at first, but with a little instruction, practice, and trust we learned to ride our bike surely and swiftly—and soon enjoyed a new-found freedom of going where we wanted.

But let's not get going too fast. If you've struggled with your weight for a long time, or if you're anxious about making changes in your life, you might be tempted to jump right into the weight-loss program in Part II. I advise you to be patient. First let yourself understand and learn the practice of self-hypnosis, at least until you feel comfortable entering and maintaining a self-hypnotic trance. It's while in trance that the drawbridge is down for suggestions to your unconscious mind. That's when to get started on your weight-loss goals.

This chapter will try to explain many of the issues that most people wonder about when first setting out to learn about self-hypnosis. It will help you understand just what self-hypnosis is, how it works, and why it's so effective.

Describing Self-Hypnosis

Before we get into the practical matters of self-hypnosis—the how, when, and where—let's try to get clear just what we're talking about. Unfortunately, self-hypnosis is hard to define because it is not a *thing* but a *process*, and so we can't say what it *is*, exactly, but we can describe what it feels like, what its effects are, and how you do it.

First, consider what self-hypnosis feels like. Have you ever had a vivid daydream? Or, have you ever been so completely absorbed in an activity—like listening to music, watching a movie, or reading a good book—that you've lost track of time, or stopped noticing what's going on around you? If you answered "yes" to either question, then you've been in a state of mind much like a self-hypnotic trance.

But with one big difference: Self-hypnosis is not wandering or aimless like a daydream; nor is it created and directed by someone else, such as an author, composer, or filmmaker. Self-hypnosis is a focused, channeled trance in which *you guide yourself* to a desired result or goal, such as stress management, pain relief—or weight loss.

Self-hypnosis feels something like meditation, calming and centering, and in fact the two have much in common. Both begin with breath work and mental imagery to relax and focus your attention; both seek to quiet the mind and have you look within as a detached observer. But if their paths are similar, their directions are very different. In meditation, the goal is simply heightened awareness or enlightenment; in self-hypnosis, *you* decide on the goal, which can be anything from awareness to stress management, to mind-body healing, to sports performance, the list goes on and on. When you're meditating you might look as if you're in self-hypnosis, but within a self-hypnotic trance you're actively goal-directed.

Because people in a trance often have their eyes closed, many assume self-hypnosis must feel like being asleep. In fact, as you might know, the Greek word "hypno" actually means "sleep." But self-hypnosis is nothing like sleep. Quite the opposite. The brain-wave patterns of people in a self-hypnotic trance show an alert wakefulness, and self-hypnosis patients often report the feeling of an active learning experience, or of a relaxing mind-body interaction in which they feel freed and empowered.

Secondly, what are the effects of self-hypnosis? The effects are wide-spread and will actually vary with different people's perspectives and objectives. It's rather like the story of the seven blind men trying to describe an elephant: Our descriptions will differ depending on what part of the beast we've gotten hold of. Still, in general, there are remarkable mind-body effects possible with self-hypnosis. By practicing self-hypnosis you can gain access to areas of yourself that are normally out of the reach of your conscious mind.

If you doubt this, sit down and passively but purposely try to slow your heart rate by ten percent, or try to raise the temperature of your hand by a degree or two. These are only minor examples of internal changes you can easily accomplish with no training at all in self-hypnosis. Once you've read this book and mastered self-hypnosis, you'll be able to make much more significant changes in *chemical*, *physical*, *psychological*, and *emotional* parts of yourself.

In the area of pain relief, for instance, major surgeries have been performed with self-hypnosis as the only anesthesia.

Take the documented case (1980) of Victor Rausch. A dental surgeon, Dr. Rausch had used self-hypnosis in his practice for years and was highly experienced and confident with trance induction. When he had to undergo gall bladder surgery, he chose to use self-hypnosis instead of any chemical anesthesia. The surgery was performed without complications and without pain.

Another dramatic physical and emotional change made possible with self-hypnosis is losing weight and keeping it off.

Julie, a thirty-five-year-old waitress, had been struggling with her weight for nearly a decade, ever since her first pregnancy. She seemed to have been on a continual diet, with no lasting results. She didn't like the way she looked. Her physician had urged her to lose weight for the sake of her health. The final straw was when she overheard two customers at work commenting about her size. At that point she began instruction in self-hypnosis, with the goal of eating less and exercising more. Julie lost sixty-five pounds in nine months. More important, two years later the extra weight was still off. She was exercising regularly and she loved the way she looked and felt. You can read Julie's whole story in Chapter 13.

Still other effects of self-hypnosis are control over fears, relief of stress, freedom from unwanted habits, resistance to disease and aging, and increased performance at work and in sports. As you can see, the life-enhancing effects of self-hypnosis are limited only by your desire to change.

And lastly, how do you do self-hypnosis? For this, you'll need to keep on reading.

So far, then, here's a definition of self-hypnosis that seems to explain the feeling and the effects of the phenomenon:

Self-hypnosis is a relaxed and focused state of mind in which positive suggestions are received and acted on much more powerfully than in normal experience.

How Does Self-Hypnosis Work?

Although no one has figured out exactly what goes on in self-hypnosis, or why it's so effective, the most satisfying theory is as follows.

While in this absorbed state of mind, two special things happen: You focus your attention much more clearly than when awake or asleep; and you also relax the critical, questioning mind that usually guides you in life. During this time of heightened awareness and acceptance, suggestions appear to go directly into the unconscious mind, where they find fertile soil for stimulating the growth of new ideas and perspectives. Thus the secret of self-hypnosis is that it takes you deep inside, and when you nurture the seed of well-being within you, letting it take root in your unconscious, it can grow and blossom in your conscious mind.

But what do we mean by the conscious and the unconscious mind? You might think of the conscious mind as the everyday, sensible, rules and regulations part of yourself—the part that wants you to keep on doing what's familiar, or what seems to have been working for you. The conscious mind is valuable, no question; it has helped you survive by making sure you learn from past experience. But it's not nearly as important as it thinks. Its center is the ego, and it's filled with exaggerated notions of self-importance.

On the other hand, you can think of your unconscious mind as the emotional, intuitive, and loving part of yourself. This is the part that wants you to see life as an adventure, to be open to new experiences, and to move toward a more creative existence. Its center might be called the "inner voice," and it is bubbling and brimming with positive human potentials.

There's no getting around it. If you want to go beyond your conditioning, programming, and upbringing—the habits and attitudes you've acquired in the course of your life—you must tap into your unconscious mind. Conscious resolutions, reminders, and self-criticism won't get you very far. The truth is, the conscious mind is only about 10 percent of your mental capacities, although the ego believes it's far more than that, more like 90 percent. In fact, it's just the opposite. The unconscious is a reservoir of 90 percent of your inner resources, and you'll find your greatest possibilities for growth and change in this vastly underutilized unconscious part of yourself.

Dr. Milton Erickson, the modern master of medical hypnosis—and my friend and mentor—was crystal clear on this point. He regarded the conscious mind as severely limited in its role in our health and well-being. He said the unconscious mind must be allowed through self-hypnosis to do the creative work, then the conscious mind could receive the new ideas and perspectives, and fit and focus them in our daily lives. A favorite metaphor of his was that the unconscious is the manufacturer, the conscious is the consumer, and self-hypnosis is the bridge between them.

Who Has Control in Self-Hypnosis?

A question often asked in regard to hypnosis is: Who's in control, you or the hypnotist? And the unasked question is: Can you be made to do something against your will? Of course, in *self*-hypnosis you are in control of your own trance, and so such considerations are not even an issue. You will always be giving yourself positive, constructive suggestions.

And yet there remains for many people an uneasiness about giving up their conscious control, a fear of being taken over by someone else's will, which, sadly, has been fostered by stage hypnotism, novels, movies, and TV. This is called the "Svengali Effect," after the early film, *Svengali* (1931), in which a bearded madman (played by John Barrymore) hypnotized young women to do his bidding and commit crimes for him. But even very recent films and television shows depict hypnosis as the tool of evil geniuses. And certainly stage shows featuring hypnotism strike fear in people's hearts that they can be made to act foolishly or do something they wouldn't do otherwise—maybe quack like a duck, croon like a lounge singer, or laugh uncontrollably.

However, when you watch stage hypnotists, you should realize that they're showmen using tricks to entertain an audience and to deceive people into believing that the hypnotist is all-powerful. First, by asking for volunteers the hypnotist gives the participants tacit permission to leave their inhibitions offstage. Then the group is assured that they're not responsible for their actions—after all, they've been hypnotized. The hypnotist also promises love and approval (in the form of applause and laughter) from the audience if the participants do the outrageous. And last they put subtle but powerful pressure on each volunteer not to "spoil the show." With all of these positive and negative reinforcements, it doesn't really matter whether the participants are hypnotized or not. They're fully primed to do foolish and fantastic things. Let the show begin.

Fiction aside, the truth is that there is no relinquishing of volition with hypnosis, no being controlled against your will. While I recommend that you *never allow an unqualified person to use hypnosis with you*, research has shown that people will follow only those hypnotic suggestions that are in their fundamental interests. In fact, many studies show that subjects under deep hypnosis will ignore a command to act against their own best interests—and will come out of trance if pressed to comply. A hypnotherapist might help to guide or develop your trance, but you are always in control.

It's also important to realize that self-hypnosis actually allows you *more* self-control rather than less. In practicing my own self-hypnosis, and in more than twenty-five years of teaching thousands of individuals, I've discovered that when you learn to let go of some of your conscious control, you gain a powerful sense of freedom in your life. It's *your* unconscious mind, don't forget, and when you've empowered it through self-hypnosis, you can count on it to protect you and care for you when you're awake or asleep, dreaming or meditating, relaxing or in hypnotic trance.

Who Can Benefit from Self-Hypnosis?

In the past, doctors who used hypnosis in their practice would routinely give their patients one of several susceptibility tests to determine their chances of success or failure. Some patients scored high and were approved for treatment; others scored low, were deemed unhypnotizable, and were offered other options.

More recently, however, studies have shown that even those who score low on these tests are indeed hypnotizable. The problem is that there are a great many variations in trance induction techniques, and so a poor score on one test means only that the person is not responsive to the particular method used in *that* test.

Now, when Dr. Erickson developed his technique of self-hypnosis, he found a method that was successful with nearly everyone, even with referral patients who had tested as "unsusceptible" to hypnosis, and who had been given up as hopeless. Many scientists and researchers in the area of hypnosis have now come to agree with Erickson that, given the right approach, practically everyone is able to enjoy the benefits of hypnosis. It's only a matter of finding the *right technique for the individual*.

Why *Self*-Hypnosis?

Dr. Erickson, as a therapist and teacher, pioneered the use of individualized hypnosis techniques to fit the unique experiences and needs of each patient. He developed an indirect, permissive, and flexible language for hypnotic suggestion, using phrases such as "You may feel . . . ," or "Perhaps you will notice . . . ," that don't command or direct the patient, but leave open the possibility of some different, more personal experience. And he also found hypnosis to be most effective when he blended his suggestions with the patient's own words, images, and symbols—the personal language of their unconscious.

Erickson was so interested in personalizing hypnosis because, as he said many times, he knew that "all hypnosis is self-hypnosis"—that it's always a do-it-yourself job. This means that only *you* have the power to hypnotize yourself, or to be hypnotized by someone else. The power is yours, not the hypnotist's. This also means that no one else heals you; a doctor or therapist might help you learn how to heal yourself, but the healing comes from you.

I follow this philosophy in my private practice, and also in this book.

Thus you'll find the book offers you the choice of a number of methods of entering and deepening your self-hypnotic trance. You can find the method or methods that you're most comfortable with and that work best for you. Many readers will be successful using several or all of the methods presented; but if one or another doesn't seem right for you, feel free to try another. Also, the book will show you how to modify and adapt the methods to the uniqueness of your own personality, circumstances, and experiences.

In addition, you'll find many, many places in these pages where you're asked to blend something from your own life experiences into the trance script, or to put some of your own words into the suggestions. If you take a few moments to personalize the scene or the language, you'll reach your goals more quickly.

• • •

Most of us can remember the first time we rode a bicycle. It was a shaky but exciting experience. And yet with a little practice we soon discovered we had some control over a new dimension of our abilities—increased balance and coordination.

Of course, we already had balance and coordination in things like running and playing. But this was something special, a delightful enhancement of our natural skills that gave us the means of dramatically expanding our boundaries.

This delightful personal expansion is what you can expect when you learn the skill of self-hypnosis. The journey awaits.

CHAPTER 2

Practical Questions

As your eagerness to start practicing self-hypnosis grows, you more than likely have some questions about the practical matters of where, when, how long, and so forth. I'll try to answer these important basic questions now.

Where Should I Practice Self-Hypnosis?

Some people can relax nearly anywhere—and relaxation is the starting point for all self-hypnosis. If you're one of these people, you'll likely find that you can practice self-hypnosis wherever you like. Most of you, however, will want to find a quiet, private place for your first sessions.

In today's world it's hard to escape noise and other outside distractions, but do your best to select a place as quiet and personal as possible. Later, when you're comfortable entering a trance easily and quickly, you'll be able to use outside sounds and disturbances to relax even more. You'll be able to do your self-hypnosis while sitting in a theater before the movie starts, while relaxing in your airline seat, or while waiting in your dentist's office. Almost anywhere. For now, though, try to find a place that's as silent and peaceful as possible.

If you choose an outside site, it should afford you privacy.

Better a secluded backyard than a front porch where someone might bother you. When you're a bit more experienced and comfortable entering trance, you might enjoy practicing in the warmth and freshness of a sunny day at the beach, or sitting in a park.

Indoors will usually be better for most of you to begin with. A bedroom, sewing room, den, or study might best suit you— especially if you have children. If it's hard to find privacy in your home, try sitting in your parked car. Or if you're at work, close your office or classroom door during your lunch hour. Do the best you can and, if possible, keep the lighting subdued.

Most importantly, the place should be as *comfortable*, *safe*, and *free* from interruptions as you can find.

When Should I Practice?

Taking time to practice is essential to developing your skill in self-hypnosis. It's helpful to recognize that the time you give to your trance work is like gold you deposit in a bank for making positive self-change. Both the amount and the quality of time you invest create the value of your experience.

But there is no set timetable for everyone. Most of you will probably do better with a regular schedule for your self-hypnosis; but some might want to allow for variation and spontaneity in their practice times. You decide.

If a regular time sounds right, you might find that early morning is the best time for you to practice self-hypnosis. It's often a quiet time in the house when you can gather your thoughts before the day's rush and scatter.

Or you might discover that midday is an ideal time in the cycle of your day to take a trance break. Whenever your midday occurs, it's a rest point between morning and evening, and a time both to review the morning's experiences and to prepare for the balance of the day.

Or you might find that bedtime is your best time for self-hypnosis, a time to breathe and let go of the day's stress, helping you relax for a good night's sleep.

On the other hand, if your life doesn't follow a daily schedule, or if you're the sort of person who can't stand routine, you might find you prefer to do your self-hypnosis when the occasion presents itself. It doesn't really matter when. Remember, your self-hypnosis is an investment in self-care, and the important thing is that you don't put off your practice time and short-change yourself.

How Long Should I Spend Practicing?

As for how long to spend on self-hypnosis, a good rule of thumb is to allow yourself about twenty to thirty minutes for your first trance sessions. Some of this time will be spent relaxing and putting yourself into trance. Be patient. As you practice and become more skilled at entering trance, you'll probably find you need only eight or ten minutes for an effective session. Eventually, the majority of your self-hypnosis time will be spent working on suggestions and visualizations for specific goals and changes.

In general, the more work you want to do with yourself, and the more complex your goals, the longer you'll need to spend in trance. Still, many people focus on having only five-minute self-hypnosis sessions, several times a day. Repetition is a successful strategy, and the trance-entry practice you get will make it even easier to return again and again for quick relief.

In other words, the timing is up to you. At first you might prefer long trance sessions that are extremely engrossing and stimulating. Then again you might come to find that brief, focused, repetitive trance and suggestion techniques work best for you. And certainly blending both of these and other sorts of trances can also prove valuable.

One other point. Some people learn self-hypnosis quickly and others take more time. The speed with which you learn self-hypnosis has nothing to do with how successful it will be for you once you've mastered it. Your unconscious is on your side and will be patient as you absorb this knowledge at your own pace.

Should I Sit or Lie Down?

Most people find that a relaxed sitting position for self-hypnosis is better than lying down. Lying down makes it easy to drift off to sleep when you're in a very relaxed state of mind. Of course, if going to sleep is your goal with that session, then lying down is fine.

Select a comfortable chair with a back that gives your head some support, or that allows you to sit upright. If your head is unsupported when you relax, it will likely roll back even more. This can become uncomfortable after a few moments, or can even startle you out of your trance. A pillow might help.

Your chair may have armrests or not. Place your arms at your sides or on the arms of the chair if that's more comfortable, or let them relax in your lap. The most important thing is to be *comfortable*.

Should I Have My Eyes Open or Closed?

It really doesn't matter if you keep your eyes open or closed in self-hypnosis. Again, whatever makes you feel comfortable is best.

Most people naturally seem to close their eyes when relaxing, probably because of the fatigue in their eyelids. So, for most of you, having eyes closed is the easier way to begin learning self-hypnosis. However, many people skilled in self-hypnosis prefer to enter and stay in a trance with their eyes open.

If you wish to keep your eyes open, you might want to fix your gaze upon some spot that has slow and regular movement, or no movement at all. Concentration is vital in developing and maintaining your trance, and visual distractions such as busy people, traffic, or television can disturb you. You might wish to experiment with an eyes-open trance to see how it works for you.

Either way, the experience of self-hypnosis is the experience of seeing with the mind's eye, watching scenes and images that play out on your own internal movie screen far more clearly and vividly than in normal life. Borrowing a phrase from an intriguing movie title, you'll be seeing with your "eyes wide shut."

How Do I Get the Most Out of This Book?

There's an old story about a young man rushing down the street with a violin case under his arm. He frantically stops an old gentleman and asks, "How do I get to Carnegie Hall?" The old man looks at the impatient young man and somberly replies, "Practice, practice, practice."

The journey to self-hypnosis requires a little knowledge, and a lot of patience, commitment, trust . . . and practice. But the benefits are enormous and can positively affect everything you do.

And it can work for everyone.

The next six chapters will teach you the skills and take you through the basic steps in learning self-hypnosis—and will give you plenty of techniques to practice to get you started on the road to *your* ultimate goal.

CHAPTER 3

Plans and Preparations

Before setting off to explore a foreign country for the first time, most of you would want to make a few basic plans and preparations. You'd want to have a good idea of where you were going and what stops you were making along the way. You might also want to know a little of the language, to be able to get around more effectively. And you'd want to be sure your vehicle had plenty of power to get you to your destination.

All of these are also true for the self-hypnosis journey. Effective self-hypnosis actually begins before you settle down in your chair, relax, focus, and enter your trance. First you need to think through your goals for your self-hypnosis; then you need to learn some of the language of the unconscious; and last you need to check to make sure your motivation is on full.

Setting Specific Goals

Before beginning your first self-hypnosis session, take a few minutes to write down your goals in a notebook or journal. What do you want to achieve with self-hypnosis? Where exactly do you want to this work to take you?

This might sound unnecessary—you want to lose weight, right?—but you need to examine your goals carefully to make sure that they're as clear and specific as possible. Giving yourself detailed, well-defined goals is vitally important. Trying to work toward vague or hazy objectives can be like trying to see over the horizon through foggy binoculars. The clearer and more focused your goals, the more quickly and easily you'll see positive changes.

For instance, the goal to "lose weight" is certainly accurate, but it's far too general; even the goal of "eating less" might be too broad to be effective. You'll do better with a more specific and personal objective. Try to spell out in detail what losing weight would be like for *you*. Try to find specific instances showing you being thinner or lighter. Try to think of real situations in which you can demonstrate a new attitude toward food. Maybe you'd enjoy fitting easily into smaller clothes, or feeling yourself running effortlessly on the beach. Maybe you can imagine eating smaller portions at your favorite restaurant, or turning down that favorite between-meal snack.

Think up examples of your own, but the important thing is to make your goals as specific as possible: *I will feel full with one portion of food at my mealtimes, three times a day, at eight, one, and six o'clock.* Always try to give your unconscious mind the clearest picture you can of what you want to accomplish.

One Small Step at a Time

While some goals are too general to be a clear target, some are also too big to be reached effectively. Even specific, well-described goals might be unattainable if you know deep down you're taking too big a leap.

Generally speaking, your self-hypnosis will be more effective if you approach your goals in smaller, intermediate steps, one modest success leading to the next. Particularly if your goals are ambitious, you're better off making steady, gradual progress, one step at a time. Most of us can't drive a spike into a plank with one mighty blow, but we can do the job with many repeated taps. So it is with self-hypnosis. Seldom are there instant remedies.

Suppose your goal is to lose eighty pounds that you've been carrying around for a long time—say, eight years. This situation is not uncommon.

And yet, if you set "eighty pounds" as your overall weight-loss goal, you'll likely be setting yourself up for disappointing results. Eighty pounds is a great deal of weight, and it's been a part of you for a long time. Adding a reasonable time limit for your weight loss—"this year" or "by summer"—is a step in the right direction, but is still too vague to be very effective.

A better idea is to approach your long-range goal of eighty pounds in specific increments of achievement. Try making your intermediate goal three pounds a week, or maybe fifteen pounds in eight weeks. These are objectives you can reach—they're "doable"—and then you can build from there with another series of steps.

A bonus is that you'll enjoy the satisfaction of your small successes, which will strengthen your resolve to achieve the next goal. In this way, cycles of accomplishment replace cycles of disappointment and failure that usually accompany trying to do too much too soon with a long-standing problem. (Note: with major weight loss, it's always important to ask your physician's advice on what's safe for a person in your physical condition.)

Whenever you create specific, personalized, attainable goals, you give your unconscious mind a clear and credible target to shoot for. At the same time, your successes show your *conscious* mind the rewards of putting time and effort into your self-hypnosis program. This will help you keep practicing. And remember: Self-hypnosis only works for you when you work at it.

Imagery: The Language of the Unconscious

The language of the unconscious is the language of imagery. So if you want to communicate effectively with your unconscious mind, you'll need to learn a little bit about using imagery to set and describe your goals.

What's imagery? An image is simply a mental picture of something. Close your eyes and remember what you had for breakfast. Or describe what your front door looks like. Or your favorite pair of shoes. In order to tell me any of these things you had to remember them and picture them in your imagination. This is imagery. "The soul never thinks without a picture," said Aristotle.

But imagery is not only visual. Imagery also conjures up smells, textures, sounds, and tastes. Can you recall what it feels like to walk barefoot on the beach? Or what a wood fire smells like? Or what chocolate tastes like? If you're really hungry, your mental image of a favorite meal may be so vivid that you can nearly smell and taste the food as you imagine it. Your mouth might even water at the thought, and your mood brighten.

Because imagery—a creation of the mind—can call up strong physical and emotional responses in this way, it's a powerful tool in self-hypnosis. It seems that, while you're in trance, mental pictures enter your unconscious mind much more readily and completely than abstract words. So by using imagery you're able to speak with greater clarity and richness to your unconscious, and thus develop a deeper level of communication. In self-hypnosis, a mental picture is worth pages and pages of verbal suggestions.

Learning the Language

You'll need to "speak" with imagery from the very first time you practice self-hypnosis. It's an integral part of learning to relax and to focus your attention inward as you enter a trance state. Now, all of us have the ability to communicate with imagery, but not all of us have developed much proficiency with the language. So let's take some time at this point to sharpen up your imagery skills.

Here is a variation of some imagery exercises devised by Dr. Michael Samuels and Mary Samuels:

1. Gaze at one of the geometrical shapes below. Then shut your eyes and try to visualize it.

2. Examine for a few moments a three-dimensional object in your home or workplace, such as an orange, a glass of water, or a lamp. Again, close your eyes and imagine the object.
3. Visualize a schoolroom from your childhood.
4. Visualize your house or your apartment, room by room.
5. Visualize a person you know, from the front and the back.
6. Visualize your own reflection in a mirror.

Practice these exercises for a few minutes every day for three or four weeks, even after you've begun with your self-hypnosis. It won't take you much more time than it takes to read these directions. You might be surprised and pleased at how vivid and creative your imagery can become. You'll also be opening up a direct line of communication with your unconscious mind.

Expand these exercises with different places and objects as you increase your imaging skills. Feel free to experiment with your favorite sights, colors, and smells and sensations of touch, heat, and cold.

Personalize Your Imagery

The most powerful imagery for your unconscious is imagery that comes from within *you*—called up from all your personal memories and experiences. When you read examples of imagery in this book, feel free (in fact, you're encouraged) to change them to suit yourself.

For example, if you're suggesting to yourself that your arm is feeling cold and numb, picture a time in your life when you really did feel cold and numb. Perhaps you'll remember being in a snowball fight without gloves. Or you might recall dipping your hand into a cold mountain stream.

If you're suggesting a floating feeling in your arms or legs, find an image from your own life that calls to mind a floating experience. Perhaps you'll picture a swan floating serenely on a calm lake; puffy dandelion seeds being carried on the wind; or the sensation you had of floating on an inner tube or a small raft.

The important thing is to create images from your own experience. Use the suggestions in this chapter only to stir your memories for images that are yours alone. You never need share or reveal your images. So be creative, and allow the positive images to flow from your mind as freely as the wind blows. Fill your images with colors, sounds, aromas, textures, and tastes. Become absorbed in your images and allow them to seem as real to you as you can.

Your success with self-hypnosis will increase as you become better at using imagery—the language of your unconscious mind—to place requests for change.

Symbols: The Language of Suggestion

There's another language in self-hypnosis closely related to imagery. This is the language of symbols, and learning a bit of it is important because it ties your imagery even more directly and effectively to your goals.

What's a symbol? It's anything—either perceived or imagined—that represents or suggests something else. For example, a sunrise might symbolize hope or new beginnings. A dog might represent loyalty or protection. And a human heart might stand for love or courage.

Although symbols can be common, everyday things, they'll not suggest the same thing to each of you. They'll most likely have a special meaning that depends on your unique experience of life, and on the personal memories and associations you attach to them. Take the ocean. To a fisherman the ocean might symbolize bounty; to a marine biologist, evolution; to a surfer, challenge; to a Jungian psychologist, the unconscious mind itself.

Whatever they mean to you, symbols are indispensable in self-hypnosis because they stimulate your unconscious mind to do its best problem-solving. If you can speak this language of symbols a little, you can communicate your goals to your unconscious mind using your most vivid images, thoughts, sensations, and memories.

You see, in self-hypnosis, the words used to express a suggestion are less important than the associations—the mental images or feelings—that attach to the words. Leaves falling as the season turns can represent the shedding of problems, or can symbolize the changes you want to make in your life. An image of industrious ants marching quietly along the ground can be a metaphor for more productive concentration at work.

Creating Symbols

When you pause to write down your specific goals before a self-hypnosis session, see if you can also write down several symbolic images for each goal. Seize this opportunity to plunge into your creative mind and surprise yourself with the symbols you find there. Your rewards for your efforts will be like the beautiful flowers from a garden that you've planted, tended, and brought to bloom.

Below are some examples that might help you develop your own suggestion symbols. Put them in your own words and use images from your own experiences and memories. Be as creative and imaginative as you want to be.

> *Rain softly washing away pain, stress, and self-doubts.*
>
> *Turning on and off a light switch can be like starting and stopping a craving for food.*
>
> *The tea pot lets off steam when the pressure builds up, just as you can let off pressure or stress by exhaling slowly.*

Are you getting the idea?

> *A flock of birds gliding, winging toward their destination is like you soaring toward your goals.*
>
> *Water flows briskly from the bathtub faucet in a soft but steady stream, just as your positive energy flows.*
>
> *Bees can choose which flower to alight on, and you can choose which dishes you'll eat at dinner.*
>
> *With clock-beat regularity, the sun and moon and stars regulate themselves in a natural cycle, just as you can regulate your eating habits.*
>
> *In its eagerness for growth, a flower opens and blossoms, just as you can grow and blossom with more freedom from your fears.*

Now you're really getting the hang of it. Spend a few moments finding new material for comparisons and metaphors. Imagine scenes in your own way—make it as real as possible.

Remember to make your suggestions specific. The more detailed and familiar the suggestion is, the more readily your unconscious will act upon it. For example, a general and vague suggestion such as *I will concentrate my attention, I will narrow my focus*, might be accepted by the unconscious, but without a more detailed picture it may have difficulty knowing when to concentrate, or how much to focus. A more specific suggestion would be:

> *While I sit reading and studying, my mind will be focused on the words and ideas in my book. Just as a funnel concentrates and directs a flow of water, my eyes can focus and channel my concentration on the words and ideas I'm reading.*

The more specific and metaphorical your suggestions, the more force they have.

Also, make sure you find several suggestions for the same goal. Even suggestions with Pulitzer Prize–winning symbols need to be reinforced with three or four different suggestions to your unconscious mind. You might have negative associations to certain words or metaphors, creating roadblocks you might not even be aware of. Therefore, the more suggestion symbols you can offer yourself, the more likely you are to create the catalysts for the changes you desire.

Personalize Your Symbols

Try to find suggestion symbols from your own work, hobbies, memories, or even dreams. As with your imagery, the more rich and graphic your symbols, and the more personal, the more effectively your unconscious mind will understand them—and act on them.

Consider for a moment Sally, an office worker who plays guitar to relax at home and to entertain her friends and family.

Sally might calm herself and enter self-hypnosis using a common suggestion symbol such as: *I'm unwinding like a clock spring.* But perhaps a more effective suggestion for her would be: *My body releases tension and stress just as the strings on my guitar slacken when I turn back the keys.* How much more effective it is for Sally to visualize this familiar guitar image in her mind and associate it with her relaxing free time.

Again, the material for creating your personalized suggestions is all around you—in your home, in your yard, in the weather, on your street, at work, at play, in books and magazines. For instance, the next time you drive down the street, notice the wind blowing the trees or shrubs. That can symbolize the refreshing winds of change you can bring to your life. Your foot on the accelerator can represent the power you can have over your eating habits. And the road you're traveling can suggest the remarkable journey you're taking with self-hypnosis.

Making Positive Suggestions

One other important point about language: Try to make your suggestions in self-hypnosis as positive as possible.

Most people react poorly to "No" or "Do Not" statements. You can probably attest to that from your own experience. From childhood on you've heard many more "No's" than "Yes's" and you've likely developed an automatic opposition to such negatives. Which request would you be more likely to follow: "Do not close the door," or "Would you leave the door open?"

The point is that, in self-hypnosis, a negatively worded self-suggestion has a smaller chance of being accepted.

I will not eat dessert any more is a negative statement that might easily be ignored by the unconscious mind. A more effective suggestion would be a positive (and more specific) statement leading to a positive result; for example, *As I eat less and less ice cream and candy, I feel healthier and more satisfied with myself.*

Wherever you can, then, connect a positive suggestion with a promising outcome. Learning to speak to your unconscious mind in positive images and symbols will help your suggestion become adopted into action.

Of course, at first it will probably seem hard to eliminate the "No's," "Not's," "Will Not's" and other negatives from your suggestions. Relax; you'll get better with practice. Besides, a few "Never's" and "Not's" creeping in here and there are harmless if you're balancing them with plenty of "I Will's," "I Can's," "I May's," and "Perhaps Today's."

Checking Your Motivation

No matter how specific, imaginative, and positive you are in your goal-setting, however, there's one more important factor to check before starting on your self-hypnosis: Your motivation to succeed.

Motivation is a primal force that floods—or drips—into your every action. If your motivation is high, you can rise early in the morning and jog a few miles before breakfast. If it's not so high, you can easily find excuses to stay in bed a little longer and then stumble into the shower. Motivation is what makes your self-hypnosis dynamic in achieving goals and changes. Very simply, the more motivated you are to lose weight, or to work toward any other goal, the more successful you'll be. Guaranteed.

Why? Because the greater your motivation toward a goal, the more open your unconscious mind will be to the positive suggestions you're giving it during self-hypnosis. You can't fool your unconscious mind very easily. If you aren't deeply committed to making a change, your unconscious will know. Your unconscious mind knows you best, and it won't be moved by half-hearted suggestions.

Building Your Motivation

It's likely that you're already interested in making a change in your eating habits and your weight, or else you wouldn't be reading this book. But mere curiosity or wishful thinking won't be enough to see you through. You need to have a strong desire to change, and a good way to build your motivation is by better understanding *why* you want to change. Try to answer this question: How will my life be better when I've achieved my goal?

To help with the answer, write down on a piece of paper a list of your reasons for wanting to change your life. As always, try to be as detailed and specific as possible. Since your goal is to lose weight, you might list the following reasons:

Why Lose Weight?

1. Look more attractive.
2. Relieve emotional pain.
3. Improve sex life.
4. Fit into fashionable clothes.
5. Have more friends.
6. Have more energy.
7. Feel better about myself.

No one else will see this list, so write down all your reasons, even those you think small, unimportant, or even silly. Often a reason that seems trivial to your ego can turn out to be very important to your unconscious, and by bringing it out in the open, you might find out it has more influence than you thought. Almost always in this exercise people make some surprising discoveries about their motivations and reasons for change.

Study your list and rank the items in the order of their importance to you. You can profit as well from writing down your ideas and feelings about each reason. Look at your list several times a day to remind yourself why you want to reach your goal. Strive to remain positive in your outlook. Dwelling on thoughts of doubt or failure can undermine your best intentions.

Becoming more aware of all your reasons for working on a goal increases and strengthens your motivation toward it. Also, more awareness helps you identify and dissolve any blocks of resistance to change you might have.

Unblocking Your Motivation

It's important to clear any blocks or obstacles from the path of your motivation. Often the very behaviors you want to change are firmly embedded in your daily routines and self-image. Your conscious mind might want to make changes for ego reasons, but your unconscious mind might have reasons of its own for keeping things as they are. For instance, suppose you want to stop overeating to lose weight. That might be a sincere desire at a conscious level. But unconsciously you may be overeating for an emotional reason. Or you may be getting some unconscious payoff for keeping the weight on.

One of the best ways to break through unconscious blocks is simply to give yourself permission to become aware of the reasons for holding on to your behavior. Accept the block just as it is, even without knowing exactly *what* it is. Accept that some part of yourself could want to block you from achieving your goal. Respect that there is a reason for the blockage. Self-protection from something emotionally intense might well be the reason.

I'll be explaining more about these unconscious blocks to weight loss, and how to use self-hypnosis to break through them, in Chapter 9. For now, just try to be honest with yourself—

honesty is also a motivator. By being honest and non-judgmental with yourself about your reasons for *not* wanting to achieve a goal, you can better understand your unconscious resistance, and maybe cut loose any hidden anchors that might be holding you back.

Expect Results

As your goals become more focused, your language skills improve, and your motivation increases, you'll be packed and ready to start on the road to self-hypnosis. As you journey inward, you'll be seeing new parts of yourself, hearing new (though familiar) voices, and experiencing fresh, creative thoughts and feelings. You'll also be seeing wonderful changes begin to take place. This in itself can be frightening.

Just remember that change is a natural part of existence. The seasons and the tides change. All animals and plants grow and develop. Stars are born and wheel through the night sky. Cells in our bodies divide and are replaced. Even rocks crumble and turn to sand over time. It has been said that change is the only constant in the universe.

Change is part of nature, and also part of your own nature. Milton Erickson told me many times that "Everyone is an individual in a process of development." Use self-hypnosis to help guide that development—let it be the vehicle that carries you to your goal. Set your expectation right now that you will see the results you want from your self-hypnosis.

CHAPTER 4

Breathing and Relaxing

The research has been done, the questions answered, the preparations completed. Now it's time to get started on the journey to self-hypnosis.

In this chapter you'll learn the first steps to self-hypnosis, simple and effective ways to quiet your mind and body and to focus your attention on your innermost thoughts, feelings, and experiences.

So, get comfortable in your quiet, personal place, and settle into your favorite chair. Let's begin.

Healthy Breathing

In self-hypnosis, the first thing you need to do is relax, fully relax, and the fastest and easiest way to relax that I know of is to pay attention to your breathing. Turn your attention inward: What's your breathing like right now? If it's quick and shallow, then you're probably a little tight inside, a little stressed. For most of us, this is normal, everyday breathing—short and rapid breaths, with the chest expanding and contracting, and the stomach held a little flat.

But there's a much healthier way of breathing. It's a technique taught by yoga masters from ancient times to help people develop internal calm and tranquility.

This healthy breathing is what I like to call "belly" breathing, the deep, slow abdominal breathing that comes from the healing center of you. Try taking some belly breaths. As you slowly inhale through your nose, feel your belly rounding outward and your diaphragm stretching as your lungs fill with air. Hold for a second or two. Then exhale through your mouth and feel your belly moving in and your diaphragm relaxing as your lungs deflate. Don't be concerned with the appearance of your stomach or the sound of your exhaling breath. This breathing is for your health.

Slow, full, rhythmic breathing of this sort triggers what Dr. Herbert Benson called a "relaxation response," automatically lowering your heart rate, increasing your blood flow, and relaxing your muscles. You'll find that you can do this kind of breathing anywhere, anytime you feel tense and pressured. Experts in relaxation like Dr. Benson recommend that you take at least forty of these deep abdominal breaths every day.

If you do nothing more with self-hypnosis than learn to belly breathe for relaxation, your life will be healthier, and you will feel stronger, more filled with energy, more vital, and more alive.

But healthy breathing has another wonderful function: It's also the starting point of a self-hypnotic trance.

Breathing into Self-Hypnosis

The best way to start your self-hypnosis sessions is by taking several extra slow, full belly breaths. Inhale through your nose to the count of four, letting your belly swell outward. Hold your breath for a count of four. Now exhale through your mouth to a count of four. Exhale completely; empty your lungs as if blowing up a balloon. Wait a few seconds, and begin again. Try to take at least four or five of these of these healthy belly breaths before entering a trance. That's all there is to it.

Notice that breathing is a cycle with both an activating phase and a relaxing phase. A deeply inhaled breath is activating—oxygen stimulates the brain and feeds the cells throughout the body. Exhaling is the letting go—tension is released, carbon dioxide is expelled, and the muscles naturally relax.

The details are important. Inhaling through your nose keeps your throat from drying out. Holding your breath for four beats helps you avoid feeling lightheaded from the increased oxygen levels in your brain. And exhaling through your mouth lets you slow down the release of air for the full four counts.

The timing, however, is flexible. As you practice with the healthy breathing cycle you might want to hold your breath an extra beat, or make the exhale double that of the inhale. Find a comfortable rhythm for you. If you do start to feel a little dizzy, stop for a while before continuing. Also, you don't need to breathe so deeply that your lungs burn. The whole experience should be soothing and relaxing.

Observe Your Turning Points

You might want to deepen your relaxation response with a simple breath-awareness exercise. First, concentrate your attention on your breathing. With your eyes open or closed, put your hands on your belly and focus on your body movements as you inhale and exhale. Do this for about a minute to slow yourself down, or until you can observe your breathing as a continuous flow through your thoughts, feelings, and images.

Now turn your attention to the turning points in your breath cycle, the moments when your inhale becomes an exhale, and vice versa. Wait for these turning points and simply observe them. Do this for two or three minutes, or more. By watching and feeling these moments of transition, giving them your total attention, you'll find yourself relaxing more fully than ever before. You'll also be amazed to find yourself feeling friendly and accepting toward your breathing—and toward yourself as a whole person. All you have to do is become aware of the turning points in your breathing. It might be helpful to imagine waves on the beach rolling in and out endlessly. Just like your breaths. Enjoy the feeling and the movement as you get ready to enter your trance.

Progressive Relaxation: Active

"An anxious mind cannot exist within a relaxed body," said Edmund Jacobson (1964). Jacobson designed a number of "progressive relaxation" exercises—both active and passive—to ease tensions and calm anxieties through highly focused muscle awareness. These exercises can be used in place of, or as an extension of, the breathing techniques described above.

One of Jacobson's most popular methods involves becoming aware of the tension stored in each muscle group in your body, actively exaggerating that tension, and then releasing it.

Here's how to do it. Get in a comfortable position. Start with your hands and arms. Taking a deep breath, make a fist with one hand, tighten the muscles, and feel the tension. With your eyes closed, imagine the tension in your body flowing to your fist like a stream of water or like a mild electric current. Use whatever image seems most comfortable to you.

After holding this clenched fist for a few seconds longer, relax the muscles of your hand as you slowly exhale. At the same time, visualize your tension, stress, and anxiety disappearing like smoke in a breeze.

Next, extend an arm in front of you, spreading your fingers as wide as possible, and arching your wrist and fingers upward as if waving goodbye. Keep your arm and fingers rigidly extended for eight to ten seconds, as you slowly inhale.

Slowly exhale and gradually relax the muscles in your fingers, hand, and arm, and then lower your arm to rest at your side. Feel the difference between the muscle tension before the exercise and after.

Do the exercise again with that arm. Then, repeat the process with your other arm. Or do both arms at the same time. Do the exercise as slowly as you can; the slower you go, the more effective it is.

Follow the same procedure with your feet and legs; back, abdomen, and chest; shoulders, neck, and facial muscles. Work one group at a time, from top to bottom, or the reverse. Curl your toes and hold; tense your calf and thigh muscles and hold; tighten your stomach, flex your chest, shrug your shoulders, rotate your neck, open your mouth and eyes wide in surprise, furrow your brow, clench your jaw—and hold. With each group, one after the other, slowly inhale as you tighten your muscles rigidly, hold your breath for a few seconds as you maintain the tension, then release it along with your breath, feeling the tension float or melt away.

To begin, do each muscle group twice, and repeat with specific groups as often as you wish to relax more deeply or release more tension. For instance, your shoulders, neck, and facial muscles store a great amount of tension. Pay special attention to these areas. Allow any accumulated worries or anxieties to fall away like leaves falling from a tree in autumn.

With some practice, you'll be able to work up or down your body pretty quickly. Also, after a few months, you might not need to go through all the muscle groups each time you sit down for self-hypnosis. But if you're feeling tense and unable to focus your attention easily, this *active* progressive relaxation can do wonders.

Progressive Relaxation: Passive

Jacobson also developed an effective *passive* progressive relaxation technique. This requires no muscle tensing at all, but uses the natural feelings of relaxation you've experienced at one time or another in different areas of your body. This is a more private, internal exercise, and is easy to do in a quiet, peaceful setting, perhaps while lying on the grass at a park, or while sitting in the sun on a lake shore or at the beach.

Begin by taking several deep, satisfying breaths. Close your eyes and imagine your tensions flowing out of your body with each breath you exhale. Do this for three or four breaths. Allow any thoughts or worries to enter your mind, but direct them out with each breath. Imagine troubling thoughts as a current of water that can be channeled out of you as you slowly exhale.

After a few moments, begin focusing your attention on your toes. Think about how they feel. Think about the walking you've done today and about how your feet and toes can now rest. Imagine the tension and pressure of walking or running as draining out, flowing out of your feet.

Next try visualizing the flow of tension running down your calves. Feel the flow draining out of you like water out of a drain spout, or like warm syrup out of a bottle. Find images that you can visualize clearly.

Move up your legs and continue your slow deep breathing. Imagine your legs as large rags that are wet and limp. Feel your legs get heavy and relaxed.

Stay with this relaxation process, moving up through your buttocks, stomach, back, and chest. Feel the heaviness in your stomach as the muscles let go of the tension. Let the sinking feeling spread throughout your abdomen.

Allow any tension to gather and flow down your arms. Let it drain from your head and face, and, like melting wax, flow down your arms and hands and out of your fingers.

Roll your head from side to side and feel the tension breaking loose and flowing down and out. Take a deep breath and, as you exhale, feel your arms and hands heavy with the flow of residual tension. Feel the tension melting and draining out of you like warm butter. Imagine squeezing out the last bit of tension and stress from your shoulders down to each finger.

After another deep breath, go back over your entire body and search for any remaining tension. Examine your forehead, jaw, and neck. Carefully imagine stress and tension draining out of your back, buttocks, and genital areas. If there is any place you think might be trapping some residual tension, focus on it and allow it to feel warm and heavy.

Try visualizing all of your tension evaporating like alcohol in an open dish. Feel your tension dissolving like a pinch of salt in warm water. Let it be washed away.

Remember the Feeling

Whichever method you've used, breath work or body work, once you're satisfied that you feel as comfortable and relaxed as possible, take some time to examine the feeling. Describe it to yourself in as many ways as you can. You want to remember this feeling of deep relaxation.

Feel it, perhaps as a warm glow, like coals radiating heat. Or see it as a shimmering of sand in the desert sun. Imagine yourself perhaps as a color, as orange or a warm pink; picture yourself as an early morning sunrise or sunset sky . . . a nature painting.

The important thing is to find some images or experiences with which you can identify this soothing, relaxed state, so that each time you practice self-hypnosis, you can reinforce the memory-image of the feeling. Eventually, with practice, just the image in your mind can be a cue and will produce the relaxed feeling.

Also, be sure to notice and remember which parts of your body seemed to harbor the most stress and tension. Each of us has special areas that store more tension than others—often the head, neck, and lower back. Next time, work on those areas a little longer. Be sure all the muscle tension has been dissolved.

By taking a little time to care for yourself, you can learn to stop using your body as a receptacle for your tension and emotions. Healthy breathing and relaxation techniques are keys to opening doors and letting in the fresh air.

CHAPTER 5

Entering a
Self-Hypnotic Trance

There's something especially inviting about entrances. Entry-ways, passages, portals, openings. They intrigue us, even inspire us, perhaps because they hold the promise of exploring new places, of gaining new insights, of discovering new knowledge, and of having new and possibly life-changing experiences.

Entering a self-hypnotic trance is like this. It's no coincidence that the noun "entrance" can also be a verb pronounced "entrance," which means "to put into trance," or "to hypnotize." So you can walk through an entrance, or you can have an entrancing experience, and often the two go hand in hand.

In this chapter, I'll show you several classic ways to enter a self-hypnotic trance safely, easily, and comfortably. Using your keys of breathing and relaxation, you can go inside and take the first steps toward your goals of self-healing and self-change.

Eye Fixation

Once you're in a safe, comfortable position, and have calmed down with several deep, satisfying breaths—look in front of you. Find some small object or spot that interests you above your line of sight. This spot could be a mark on the wall, the tip of a plant leaf, a part of a picture, or anything that's stationary.

Focus all your attention on the spot or object—gaze at it, examine it in detail, observe it as if you've never seen it before. Continue slow, deep, belly breathing. Keep your attention on the spot and work all your thoughts toward it. Try to eliminate any outside thoughts and let go of all problems, worries, and anxieties as much as possible.

Don't worry if a stray thought or two slips into your mind now and again. No matter what your state of mind—excited, cautious, nervous, even skeptical—just observe your thoughts non-critically, let them pass through your mind, and in a few moments you'll find you've forgotten all about them. Later in this chapter I'll give you more ideas on how to handle distracting thoughts and stay focused.

Return your attention to your spot or object. Look closely, continue breathing, and notice how relaxed you're starting to feel. Begin giving yourself suggestions such as:

> *With each deep, soothing breath, I feel relaxation spreading down from my shoulders and back, down through my legs and into my toes. The more I relax, the better I feel.*

Put these suggestions into your own words if you prefer. The exact wording isn't important. If your goal—relaxation—is clear and your suggestions are positive, your unconscious will understand.

You might feel your eyes watering and blinking. Notice what your eyes are doing and give yourself suggestions encouraging them to close:

> *As my eyes focus on the spot before me, I may find that I feel tired. As my eyes water and blink, they are clearing away all worries, concerns, and anxieties. My body is relaxed and at ease, and my eyes and my mind can be just as comfortable, relaxed, and at ease.*

You might spend as long as ten to fifteen minutes with your eyes open during your first few practice sessions. Or you may find that in only a few minutes your eyes start to become tired and heavy. You decide when you want to close your eyes.

Continue with suggestions such as:

I may notice that, as my eyes stay focused on the spot I've chosen, I can decide when I want to close my eyes. Just as I decide when to go to sleep at night, I can decide when it's most comfortable for my eyes to close.

As best you can, keep a steady flow of positive mental images going to yourself. You can say the same thing in many ways. Change the words slightly or shift the order of the words. Find a variety of suggestions, but keep encouraging the same ideas: Concentrating on the spot you've chosen, relaxing, and closing your eyes.

Repetition of the suggestions and the monotony of the focus on one spot will soon make your eyes *want* to close. However, if after ten or fifteen minutes your eyes still feel wide open, don't worry, you can just close them gently.

Deepening the Trance

After your eyes are closed, continue giving yourself suggestions to deepen and generalize the feeling of relaxation spreading throughout your mind and body. Repeat your own words to yourself and focus on your inner voice. Allow your suggestions to drift from closing your eyes to feeling a deeper relaxation. These suggestions might be like those you used in progressive relaxation in Chapter 4, or like the personalized imagery you practiced in Chapter 3. So you don't have to search for words, it's a good idea to prepare several suggestions and images before you sit down to enter trance:

Unwinding my muscles like unknotting a rubber band

Muscles soft and relaxed like bread dough

Unstressed and unpressured as a deflated balloon

Here are some longer images you might script and rehearse beforehand:

> *While walking through a noisy, busy shopping mall recently, I entered a little shop tucked away in a quiet corner. I too can have a quiet, private, unhurried experience each time I practice self-hypnosis.*
>
> *I breathe smoothly and effortlessly as I relax, just as a car engine draws in fresh air and burns it smoothly and easily while idling. An engine needs time to cool down after a long haul up a steep grade, and my muscles and my mind need a period of relaxed coasting to cool down from the stresses and tensions of the day.*
>
> *I imagine a leaf floating down to a trickling stream. I watch the leaf gently rocking and falling, then drifting on the breeze toward a quiet cove where I'm alone, with no one to bother me. As I watch the leaf land quietly on the water and begin floating lazily downstream, my muscles release the stress and tension they're holding.*

Create new suggestions and images using your own experiences, interests, and memories, or from books, movies, television, and pictures from magazines that you find relaxing. Make these mental pictures as vivid and realistic as you can. Involve as many of your senses as possible. Imagine the sights of the busy shopping center or of the dappled light through the trees. Imagine the smells of the leaves, or of the fresh air. Imagine the sounds of the shoppers' voices, the purring engine, the babbling stream. Imagine the coolness of the water, the warmth of the sun, the breeze against your face.

Don't try to analyze your suggestions—let them flow. If one image doesn't seem to make sense, or is hard to picture in your mind's eye, don't worry—suggest a different one. Keep giving yourself a continuous flow of words, images, and symbols toward your goal.

The Candle Flame

You can make the eye-fixation technique more intriguing if you wish. Close off your room from outside things as much as possible. Turn off the lights, close the curtains, and make it completely dark. Light a small candle so that it's in front of your eyes. Then, without blinking, stare at the flame and just go on thinking that you're drifting into a dream. A dreamy, hazy relaxation will arise within you—just let this feeling float within you, as you go on staring at the candle, with this feeling hovering over you like a puffy white cloud.

You're flowing into a dream, you're becoming your dream, and as you do, say to yourself,

> *Dreams are coming . . . calming dreams are coming . . . I am flowing into a restfulness I have never known before. I am flowing into a dream. Dreaming is approaching. My limbs are relaxing.*

You'll soon feel a subtle change, and within a few minutes you can feel your body has become more relaxed. Any moment you can flow into your dream. The lids of your eyes get heavy and it becomes difficult to keep looking at the flame. Your eyes want to close. This means you're crossing the border. Everything is becoming relaxed and heavy as you become more dreamy, falling into a safe unconscious awareness and becoming very comfortable within yourself.

Counting

A faster and yet still highly effective trance induction method uses a counting technique. First, close your eyes and take several deep, relaxing breaths, paying special attention to the turning points. Now focus on your goal, perhaps to be more relaxed and confident, perhaps to bring pain relief, or perhaps to curb your overeating. Focus on your goal, whatever it is, think about it, maybe even picture it to yourself, and then state it to yourself so that you can feel it more intensely. Try to get the feeling for what your goal is.

In a minute, when you're ready . . . begin counting from zero to one hundred, feeling more and more relaxed as the numbers climb higher. Once you reach one hundred, take another deep breath, and simply count back down to zero. When you get to the bottom, all the way to zero, you'll be in a remarkably comfortable and creative self-hypnosis trance.

Enjoy your self-hypnosis for as long as you wish. Allow your intuition and your creativity to bubble up and help you be successful with your goal. You'll find it delightful to be able to tap into your own inner resources.

The Stairway to Self-Hypnosis

Here's a more visual variation on the counting method that makes an effective entrance to your self-hypnosis.

Visualize yourself at the top of a long spiral stairway. Perhaps you're up in the foggy heights of a mountain. There may be thirty steps leading down to the most relaxing, most comfortable place you can imagine. Maybe it's a place you're familiar with or once visited—a vacation spot, a cabin in the forest, or a camp site in a grassy meadow. Maybe it's a place you've only read about, or seen in a favorite movie. Or maybe you'd like to dream up a place. Real or fantasy, it doesn't matter.

Suggest to yourself the following picture:

> *As I take a deep, satisfying breath, I begin descending the stairway. Out of the fog and clouds of my busy day I move slowly toward a more comfortable, more relaxed place. Just as I can travel now with each step to a new place, a new experience, I may find that I'm curious about what I'll feel as I get closer to the bottom of the stairway.*
>
> *I don't need a train, an airplane, or a car to make this journey. I won't need a ticket, money, or baggage. All I need is my imagination, and I can take the steps necessary to bring me to my new and yet familiar feeling of deep relaxation.*

As you give yourself these suggestions, you may want to count down with each step, thirty . . . twenty-nine . . . twenty-eight. . . . Or you can simply visualize each step as you watch yourself descending the stairway. Either way, imagine yourself coming down slowly, step-by-step, and feel your relaxation increasing.

New Sensations

A way to focus your attention even further is by imagining a change in your body's sensations of warmth, coolness, numbness, and so on. When you can feel such physical changes, you'll know you've achieved a deep level of trance.

After you've counted down to zero, or "wound down" the stairway, direct your attention to your arm. Right arm or left arm—it doesn't matter which. Visualize it in your mind with your eyes still closed. Imagine your arm feeling cooler and cooler, or warmer and warmer—or heavier, or lighter, or more numb. Give yourself a soothing flow of suggestions to one or more of these effects.

If coolness seems pleasant, visualize cold, icy water running over your arm, and begin to feel a cool numbness in your fingers. If warmth seems pleasant, imagine the sun's rays on your arm, comfortable and relaxing. Let these feelings spread naturally for several moments. Take this opportunity to feel more open and relaxed.

Still concentrating on your arm, you'll gradually begin to notice a cool twinge, maybe a numbness, or a warm glow. Strengthen that feeling, whatever it might be, with more encouraging suggestions. Here's how you might proceed:

> *As my hand rests gently, comfortably at my side, I may notice a new feeling. I may soon feel a tingling at my fingertips. That feeling may be a cool tingling like touching the cold steel of a table. Or it may be a warm tingling like resting my hand on the warm sand of the beach or the desert.*
>
> *It doesn't matter which feeling. My hand may even feel numb. Or perhaps it will feel heavy, as if weights were pulling it downward. Or light, as if helium balloons were attached to each finger, the wrist, or the elbow. Feeling lighter and lighter, my hand may want to float up off its resting place. It's a comfortable lightness, a detached feeling, as if my arm is disconnected and wants to float up with the balloons.*

Continue to encourage the feeling to spread from one finger or part of the hand to the next. Go as far as you can with these sensations. Take your time. You might feel some change right away, or maybe not until the second or third practice session.

Soon you'll be able to develop a new sensation from your fingers to your shoulder. Your hand or arm may even feel so light it will float up and feel suspended on its own.

There is nothing mysterious about this new experience. You have simply entered a self-hypnotic trance and have created a physical sensation through suggestions to your unconscious mind. *This is self-hypnosis.*

Dealing with Distractions

A commonly asked question is, "What do I do when irritating noises or other distractions and annoyances break my concentration?" Certainly it can be difficult to stay focused when a jet booms overhead, when a garbage truck clangs and rumbles by outside, or when the dog next door starts barking. No matter how well you've secluded yourself, nature and technology can intrude on your self-hypnosis.

When this happens, you don't have to fight or try to ignore the noise or interruption. Besides, often the more you try to ignore something, the more you notice it. Instead of fighting the distraction, you can actually use it to deepen your trance. All that's required is a shift in your perception and you can reframe the interruption and make it part of your self-hypnosis.

For instance, if the noise is of passing vehicles, you can imagine how they might help you carry away your problems. Give yourself suggestions such as:

> *As the sound of the garbage truck approaches, I can place all my tensions and worries into a trash bag. When the truck stops at my house, I can pitch the bag of stress and problems into the truck to be hauled away to the dump.*

While giving yourself this suggestion, imagine your bag being swallowed up in the huge truck bed and driven away from you. Feel the relief of tension and pressure in your muscles as the sound of the engine retreats out of range.

Even though you may not yet be in trance, begin giving yourself suggestions that incorporate the distracting sounds. Mentally speak to yourself. If you're using one of the relaxation techniques, give yourself suggestions that will use the sounds to help you relax. For example:

> *The sounds of children playing and people busy with their own lives are reminders that I, too, can take time to do things important in my life—such as the time I'm taking right now for self-hypnosis.*

> *A dog barking makes me think of a beautiful park where all dogs run free, and where I'm relaxing on a rock by the lake.*

> *A clock ticking reminds me of my heart beating steadily. I can calm my heart with self-hypnosis to unwind from the hectic pace of the day.*

> *Just as a bird's song springs naturally from its breast, I can find a natural relaxation arising from within me as I breathe deeply and rhythmically.*

> *Just as the elevator in my building takes people up and down, to and from their apartments, self-hypnosis can take me up to new levels of awareness, or down into deeper states of relaxation.*

With suggestions such as these, you can use outside distractions to refocus on the trance induction you had begun.

Dealing with Thoughts

Distractions can also come from inside. For instance, people who think a great deal have trouble turning off their mind. Their thoughts can be like cars crisscrossing at a busy intersection, or like voices overlapping at a cocktail party. If you find you have so many thoughts in your head that you can't easily relax and enter a trance, try the following technique.

Focus on your thoughts. Notice how they come into your mind, stay a while, then depart. Observe how you can separate your thoughts and listen to one at a time. Identify one thought, then another, another, and so on.

Don't challenge your thoughts or reject them; don't even try to ignore them. The idea is not to create any conflict over your thoughts, but allow them, welcome them, and make them your point of focus for the time being.

Let your thoughts be and use them in a counting exercise. Start counting your thoughts. Begin at one and count up to forty or fifty—count them all. Become very good at counting your thoughts. Make sure you separate them so you don't count only one thought when there are really three bound together. Count carefully and accurately and notice how many different thoughts you have.

Then begin breathing slowly and regularly to a pattern of counting. Maybe breathing in on each thought and exhaling with a different thought. In a short while, you'll notice how absorbed you've become in the process of counting your thoughts, and you'll have experienced perhaps your first self-hypnotic trance.

Dealing with Emotions

Other people are so wrapped up in strong emotions—sadness, anger, grief, fear, and so on—that they can't use eye fixation or focused imagery. If you feel your emotional state is preventing you from entering trance by these methods, you might try one of the following induction techniques.

Start by getting as physically comfortable as you can. Find a place to be alone for a little while and close your eyes while taking several deep slow breaths. Focus on the emotion or emotions you're feeling at the present moment. Ask yourself what is happening in your life—right now—to contribute to your emotional state. Avoid judging your feelings or trying to improve them. There's no sense in trying to talk yourself out of feelings that have you in their grip.

Let's say you're tensed up with worry. Try to look carefully at your worry to better understand the feeling. See the worry as a place you're approaching—a house, say, or a cave, or a thicket of trees. Become aware of the entrance to your worry; focus on how the worry comes upon you or how you enter into the emotion.

Once inside with your worry, listen to the voice of your worry. No criticism, just observe and listen to gain more awareness. You can actually show understanding and compassion for the worried part of you. Make that part of you a friend. Then begin exiting the place of worry together.

Take several deep and focusing breaths—breathe out your worry, breathe in a cool focus on your inner friend. Take four or five deep breaths to let go and relax, and you'll find your worry has helped you enter trance.

Another technique is to go to a very special movie. Again, get comfortable and focus on your feelings. Only this time, begin to develop an image that you're sitting in a movie theater or screening room watching a scene from a movie about your own current life. You're the star of this movie, and your character is going through all the difficulties and feeling all the same emotions you are. You're also the camera operator, and you can zoom in to focus on one part or another of the action. You're even the writer of the movie script, and you can look into your main character's mind and heart, and see from his or her point of view.

Don't try to make anything happen in the movie; just observe and listen to the scenes of your present life as it is. Become absorbed in your movie and you'll soon discover you've entered a trance through this state of detached awareness.

You might need to watch your movie several times before you feel at ease using your emotions to reach a trance state. That's fine. Take your time, and when you're ready you can shift the scene of your movie toward your goal work.

Dealing with Life

Some distractions you may want to deal with more directly. These are disturbances to your trance that require a reaction from you: Your child knocking on the door, the front doorbell ringing, an itch on the bottom of your foot, a crashing sound from the kitchen.

These sorts of urgent disruptions are best dealt with directly. Answer the doorbell, the phone, or whatever, and then return to your self-hypnosis. Sometimes it can be more distracting to wonder what a noise or a phone call might be than to take a moment to find out. Also, if your nose itches at any time during a trance, by all means scratch it—then re-enter your trance.

Signs of Success

The passage from regular waking consciousness to hypnotic consciousness can be subtle. You might not even notice it the first time or two you try. Be patient with yourself.

Three clues that you've successfully achieved a self-hypnosis trance are:

1. Noticing that your breathing is full, slow, and rhythmical, and that you've reached a feeling of deep relaxation.
2. Noticing that your suggestions of coolness, warmth, numbness, lightness or heaviness have taken effect somewhere in your body.
3. Noticing a time distortion—that after your session, more or less time has passed than you thought.

CHAPTER 6

Developing Your Trance

When you're deeply relaxed and inwardly focused—in other words, when you've drifted into a self-hypnotic trance—your unconscious mind is more open and receptive than ever before to positive suggestions for self-care and self-change. Comfortably and quietly you've entered the nurturing, healing center of yourself, and you're ready to start working toward your goals.

How do you proceed? What do you picture and say to yourself during these precious minutes of inner access? There are hundreds, even thousands, of ways to develop your trances. There are activities to try, messages to deliver, people to meet, scenarios to play out, places to visit, and journeys to take—all in the deepest recesses of your imagination.

The trance scenarios presented in this chapter are varied and effective and will introduce some of my favorite techniques for helping you to explore your inner world and get the most out of your self-hypnosis. I've used all of these ideas thousands of times over the years in my practice, and they have been the most popular with my patients and students. Try them all at least once, and see which are most effective for you.

As you read through these mini-scripts, and the many others in later chapters, imagine that you're a loving, caring teacher reading a story to a totally open, receptive student. Don't try to pay attention to each word or any exact directions, but let the words flow into you like music. Absorb the ideas, and let them relax you and empower you. After you've read the scripts through a few times, you'll have learned them well enough to begin incorporating them into your self-hypnosis sessions.

You can use these scenes and scripts just as written, but you'll likely have more success if you rewrite them to suit yourself, putting them in your own words, choosing your own imagery, and making them more directed to your personal goals. (Some will be adapted specifically for weight loss in Part II of this book.)

Once you've personalized your scripts (or even if you don't), you can introduce them into your self-hypnosis in two ways. You can learn them by heart, or at least commit the basic ideas to memory and recite them to yourself in trance. Or if you wish, and feel it would help, you can record them word for word on audio cassette (particularly the longer ones) and play them during your trance. Either technique lets you move smoothly and comfortably through your self-hypnosis session, without feeling pressured to think of something in the moment.

Whichever way you work with these scripts—reciting from memory or recording onto tape—you need to take a moment and consider your tone of voice and your delivery. Your tone, your pace, your rhythm—they all need to express a feeling of loving self-acceptance and self-support. Your goal is to make your voice as self-loving and self-caring as possible, so even if you start out in your normal voice, see if you can relax your delivery as you get into the script, slowing your pace and softening your tone slightly. By the time you finish, you should be speaking in a much slower cadence and much more softly and rhythmically than when you began. This will also provide an audio cue for you to slow down and relax as you enter self-hypnosis.

Lastly, be patient with yourself as you explore these various monologues. You may need to practice several times before you feel their full benefits.

Breathing Colors

Here's a good way to take the healthy breathing you began practicing in Chapter 4 to a deeper level. Begin your session like always: Focus on your breathing, accept your breathing as it is, and then notice your turning points, from inhale to exhale, from exhale to inhale. Then, as you're watching yourself breathe, switch the experience into Technicolor:

> *I find purple is a healing color. So I breathe in purple, let it go everywhere in my body from my head to my toes, circulating, moving, and then I exhale purple as I release tension and stress. That's right. Like purple is a color cleaner working within me, I breathe it in, let it go everywhere, and then I breathe it out. So, as I'm watching my breath, I'm watching in color. What about orange? Orange is a color that makes everyone feel good; it's impossible to feel unhappy around orange. So I breathe it in, let it go everywhere inside, and then breathe it out. Now I can get playful with this and use the colors I love. For example, blue, I breathe it in and breathe it out, blue for tranquility and peace, like the rivers, like the ocean, like the sky. That's right. And as I continue going through the colors, I can mix some colors so I have combinations of colors and just continuing to watch my breath, letting the colors circulate and move everywhere inside, and then exhaling the colors.*
>
> *Now I know that anytime I see these colors in my everyday life, in a magazine, somebody's car, on a picture or flower, even up in the sky, these colors will bring me back to the feelings that I'm developing in this inner experience. So I breathe as many colors as I wish, breathe them in and breathe them out. That's right. Watching my breath is a very colorful and empowering experience. It's a present to myself.*

The Silver Thread

This is a powerful technique for helping your body relax and be more open to suggestions for self-change and self-healing. Naturally with your eyes getting heavy, and with your breathing deep and rhythmical . . .

I can visualize my spinal column and my backbone. Maybe remembering a physiology book or a book about the body and the structure of the body, I can visualize my backbone, gently curved, and in the middle of my backbone I can imagine a silver thread running down the center of it. That's right. My spinal column is the base of my whole body structure. Everything is connected to it. More so than my brain, which is merely at one end of my spinal column. And right in the center of my spine is a silver thread that I can find if I look closely enough. Seeing within is easy when we aren't afraid of our bones, or our blood, or our muscle.

If I keep focusing inside, I may feel my body is a great universe, all in itself. A brand new lightness can be realized like this, energy can flow easier, a silence can be felt, a deep relaxation can be experienced in a loving way. I just need to look inside, concentrate on my spinal column, feel the silver thread in the center of my body, and enjoy the deep relaxation. That's right. It's wonderful how going inside can create so much relaxation and so much peace.

Entrance and Exit

A very effective strategy for deepening or developing new qualities of a trance-state is to bring yourself out of trance and then quickly re-enter. Each time you leave and then return to the self-hypnotic state, you can reach a deeper level than before.

As I continue to talk to myself, soon I'm going to count from five to one, not yet, but in a few moments. And when I do, I'll find that as I get closer to one, I'll become more and more relaxed and perhaps even distant in my surroundings. I may feel as if I've traveled in an elevator or escalator to a vacation spot. A place where I can feel most relaxed.

And now I'm going to count and feel my elevator or escalator or staircase taking me down to that relaxing, comfortable place in my mind.

... 5 ... 4 ... 3 ... 2 ... 1 ... I can feel more relaxed now than before. I can feel the waves of comfort wash over me like the waves of sunlight flowing over me in summer. Perhaps I can even feel a floating sensation as if I'm in a balloon floating over a green meadow.

Now I'm going to go back up the staircase or elevator or escalator. As I count back up ... 1 ... 2 ... 3 ... 4 ... 5 ... I feel as if I'm going back up the stairway, feeling more wakeful, more alert, more aware of my surroundings with every number I count.

And when I reach the number five, I open my eyes, recognize my experience and, just for a moment, I'm aware of everything around me. Then I close my eyes again.

And as I close my eyes again, I count backward again ... 5 ... 4 ... 3 ... 2 ... 1 ... Slowly, comfortably, as I count backward and go down to the deep level, I can imagine the changes in my body from what I felt before. When I get to one, I can lift my index finger, and then slowly lower that finger down again, comfortably, to signal to my unconscious that I'm so relaxed.

And now, gradually, I move back up to a lighter, more alert, more wakeful state ... 1 ... 2 ... 3 ... 4 ... 5 ... eyes open and awake. I can become aware now of the changes from what I felt a few moments ago.

I can return again now. Moving back down ... 5 ... 4 ... 3 ... 2 ... 1 ... to a meadow or a sandy beach or maybe a mountain forest, I can travel in this state with my mind, to any state, to anywhere I choose. I can explore.

Your Seven Senses

You might use some of your first few trance sessions to help yourself improve your skills for creating effective imagery. In addition to practicing the Samuels exercises in Chapter 3, spend some trance time on the following inward journey to heightened awareness, guided by all seven of your senses:

I'm traveling to a favorite place, a place that I love, a place where I feel really comfortable, and a place that I know really well. Maybe somewhere I've been as a child, maybe somewhere I go regularly on my own. Maybe a place that I've created in my imagination and where there are mountains or a beautiful ocean or stream, or just some quiet sacred place I've created for myself.

*Now I see this place as never before, the colors, the shapes, the details, the parts, the whole. That's right. The hillsides, the greenery, maybe even see myself in this place, and don't just see with my eyes closed, but see with my whole body, let my whole body see this favorite place. Take it all in. **I am my eyes.***

*I listen to all the sounds, listen to my breathing inside, listen to the sounds outside, the birds, the wind, even the sounds that may have distracted or disturbed me in the past now actually enhance my experience. **I am my ears.***

*I smell the fragrances. The grasses, the pine trees, the ocean, the flowers, the time of day, the season. Some people say that life itself has a fragrance. **I am my nose.***

*I taste all the tastes of a picnic in my place, the food, the drink, I lick my lips and taste the saltiness, the sweetness, the moisture, the dryness. **I am my tongue.***

I feel all the textures and temperatures surrounding me, the bark of the trees, the sand under my feet, the warm sun, the cold stream. **I am my skin.**

I pay attention to my sixth sense, my intuition. What's it saying about this journey? What's it saying about my self-care and being in this favorite place creating this experience for myself? **I am my truest self.**

What's my seventh sense, my sense of humor saying? Am I feeling light and amused? Can I laugh a little with myself, about the awkwardness of learning something new? About the silly side of my problems? About the resistances that are arising? **I am my lightest self.**

And in this favorite place of mine, let all my senses be present now, see and feel, listen, smell, taste, intuit, and laugh. That's right. This is my place of power. This is my place of relaxation. And once I'm in this place, for a few moments or a few minutes, I'm giving myself a present of tranquility, of balance, of peace.

Fly Away

You can create inner scenarios that let you explore your life and free your spirit. How would you like to take yourself on a relaxing journey to an island? You'll be back in about five minutes and when you're done, you'll feel better, really good, more open, more positive, relaxed and confident. So taking several deep, satisfying breaths, you can begin your journey . . .

I'm going to travel to a beautiful island where the sun is warm, where the water is warm, where there are very comfortable and soothing trade winds. I can smell the salt from the ocean so keenly, I can almost taste it. And everything about this place is inviting. Really beautiful, really comfortable. And to get there, I'm going to have to travel by plane, and it will be a very easy journey. I sit in the plane, first class, of course, really comfortable. That's right, I put on my seatbelt and settle in. And as the plane takes off, I feel really at ease, very smooth, very comfortable. And once we're in the air, I can actually make a transition, going from feeling like a passenger in first class flying, to actually being the airplane. So there's a feeling of power, of strength, of direction.

And after just a little bit, I start to feel like I'm a cloud watching the plane, also watching the person in the plane, and yet still a cloud just floating, really at ease, and just watching the small plane on the journey with myself inside the plane. And after just a little bit, I start to feel like I'm the sky. The blue sky, watching the clouds, watching the plane, watching myself in the plane. Beautiful.

And in just a few moments, I'll be landing on this beautiful island. That's right. And as I arrive and get off of the plane, the first thing I notice is how good it feels to finish that part of the traveling and be right where I want to be. In a very soothing place, it actually feels healing. That's right. Just to be on this lovely island with these gorgeous bays, the dark mountains in the distance, the small islands farther out, the white sandy beaches just right for a pleasant walk and a picnic lunch. All the coral reefs for snorkeling, I can see them. Right from where I am.

So I start to take a walk on the beach and I feel the sand beneath my toes; that's right, the warm white sand, so beautiful, so comfortable. And I even get down to the water. It must be 75 or 80 degrees, really comfortable. And as I feel it on my toes, and my feet, and my ankles, those warm feelings from the water and the sun float right up through my body creating kind of a tingly, delightful feeling. That's right.

And the beautiful clouds create a rainbow of colors in the sky. There are all kinds of beautiful colors around me, *whether I look at the water or at the sky. I can even see a rainbow in the distance by the mountains. That's right. And I listen to the water lapping up on the shore, it's a beautiful sound, very, very healing, splashing up at my feet, trying to reach the palm trees, going right by the huts, the grass houses that people live in or stay in for a while.*

Pretty soon, but not yet, I'm going to have to return to the plane. But I want to take in as much of these breath-taking landscapes, these beautiful islands as I possibly can. I want to experience everything I'm seeing, and feeling, and smelling, and tasting, and hearing, and everything my intuition says about this place. I can come back here as often as I wish, anytime I want to.

So the time is up, that's right, I'm going to go back to the plane. I know the routine. I start off as passenger in my first-class seat, but after we take off, I become the plane. After a little bit I become a cloud watching the plane, and then the sky watching the cloud, watching the plane, watching myself. And pretty soon, that's right, I'm right back where I started, right where this all began. Feeling better, really good, more open, more positive, relaxed, and confident.

Driver's Education

Self-hypnosis works naturally to center you in time, or, in other words, to help you live in the present tense. Here's an easy way to practice being right here, right now, in the moment:

When I drive my car, I have my hands on the wheel, I look where I'm going, and I check the rearview mirror occasionally to see who's behind me. So just as in daily life, when I drive, the past is always behind me, the future is always in front of me, and I'm right here, right now, in the present, with both hands on the wheel.

Now if I go through life always thinking about the past and staring in the rearview mirror, I'll bump and crash into things all the time. The same with driving, the same with life. If I'm concerned about what's coming two miles, three miles down the road, and next week, next month, too far in the future, I forget about where I am, I make a lot of mistakes, and it's not very comfortable. So the future is always in front of me, the past is always behind me, I'm always in the present. Anytime I'm driving I can remind myself of this. And anytime in my daily life when I start to get too concerned about past things or future things, I can remember it's okay to check the rearview mirror every once in a while, but I don't want to be staring into it. And it's okay to be concerned about what's coming as long as I know it's out there, a mile, or two, or three miles out there in the future.

So here I am, in the present, the past behind me, the future in front of me. Here I am right now. And I know the more I can accept how my life is right now, the happier I'll feel, the more freedom I'll feel. This is really where it's at, how I'm doing right now.

The Second Watcher

One of the most important lessons self-hypnosis has to offer is how to see yourself from a new perspective—how to observe and listen to yourself without the usual judgments and self-criticisms. The following technique teaches you not only to watch yourself from a distance, but to watch yourself watching yourself, and in the process helps you see yourself as you really are:

I'm sitting in the fifteenth row of a darkened movie theater, that's right, in the fifteenth row, about in the middle of the theater, and when the movie comes on the big screen, I look up and I'm watching the story of my everyday life. So what do I think about the movie? How do I feel about the movie? Do I see anything going on in the movie? At home? At work? It's okay if I jump around from scene to scene, I don't have to follow any chronological order. I'm simply observing and listening to what's happening in my movie. I'm simply sitting back and seeing things from the fifteenth row.

Next, I want to imagine that I'm sitting back in the last row of the theater. Maybe about the twenty-fifth row. And from the last row of the theater, I can watch the person in the fifteenth row who has been watching the movie, who had all those impressions, and who just made all those comments. So from the last row what are my observations about the observer in the fifteenth row? That's right. I'm watching the watcher. And I can say anything I want, and I will accept anything I say. There is no right or wrong.

Now, from the last row, what are my observations about the movie? How do I feel about myself in the movie? How do I look? How are my relationships at home? How's it going at work? How's my health? So now I'm in the last row watching the big screen and it's the movie about my life. I'm comfortably removed yet still involved, and I'm able to see myself with different eyes. From the last row I can always see myself with different eyes.

Tomorrow

You can develop the Second Watcher trance many ways, to accomplish any number of goals. But for now, here's an idea to show you the possibilities.

In your trance, after moving your observer to the last row . . .

I want to focus on the next twenty-four hours and what I'd like to accomplish in the next twenty-four hours. Maybe it's something as simple as being relaxed and confident. Maybe it's something about weight loss. I just want take a few minutes to describe to myself what I want to feel in the next twenty-four hours. Maybe how I want to handle a certain situation, maybe a certain person, maybe myself. And so I watch the movie of my life as I want it to go, get a feeling for what's happening in the movie, listen to the dialogue, watch it from the twenty-fifth row, the last row of the theater, how I want things to go for the next twenty-four hours. That's right. I'm learning how to take the best care of myself possible with my abilities to see my life with new eyes.

The Mountain Climber

Here's an outdoor variation on the Second Watcher technique for gaining new perspectives:

It's easy to imagine being on a hill or a mountaintop, looking down on the valley of the town or city where I live, and just watching myself like a casual observer, in my everyday life, maybe from the time I awaken, through the morning, through the day, through the night until the time I go to bed. And what are my impressions from this height, sitting on the mountain or the hill and watching myself? That's right. I can talk to myself now, I can talk out loud, just be the observer, be the watcher on the mountain giving my impressions of myself in my everyday life. Maybe I can see myself interacting with other people in my life. I can just about hear the words, the conversations that drift up the mountain. That's fine.

But now I climb up to a higher place, the higher hill just beyond, from which point I can watch the watcher on the first hill, who's watching me in my everyday life. That's right. And from the higher mountain, I can also watch myself way down there in my everyday life. So I'm watching the watcher and I'm watching myself. Now what are my impressions, both of the watcher on the first mountain, and of myself in my everyday life? Good, good, I'm getting it.

I think I'll have some fun and create a powwow of sorts. The second watcher, the one on the higher hill, goes to the first mountain, to the watcher on the first hill, and they both climb down into my everyday life, and these three have a meeting, these three dimensions of myself, and they have a conversation about how I want things to go, about how important it is to see things from a new perspective.

And then when I'm ready, I can take the first watcher back up the first hill, then climb back up the second mountain myself and again watch the first watcher, and also watch myself down in the valley, down in my everyday life. Now what do I see? Am I seeing with different eyes?

The Committee Meeting

This extended scenario develops the "powwow" idea mentioned in The Mountain Climber above, and also takes your self-hypnosis further into the "self-acceptance" and "self-expression" phases of the journey.

And from this mountaintop, this second watcher perspective, I can look way down there in the valley, in my city, in my town, maybe I need binoculars or a telescope, I don't know. Maybe I can just see things more clearly than I've ever seen them before.

Way down there in my everyday life there's a committee meeting going on, maybe three or four, seven or eight different committee members sitting in a circle. And each of the committee members represents a different part of me, a different age and stage in my life. Maybe there's the five-year-old me, sitting next to the ten-year-old me, sitting across from the fifteen-year-old me, sitting near the twenty-year-old me. That's right. And all of these committee members represent different stages in my ability to do the best I could with my life.

So with my eyes closed and feeling more and more comfortable and open (and knowing I can go back to the mountaintop and the second watcher perspective anytime), I make my way down into the valley, down into my everyday life, down into the committee meeting, realizing how important it is to accept the different ages of myself, and to give them all a chance to express their different feelings.

As I come near the circle, within hearing, the child in me, one of the committee members, is maybe saying, "Be more playful, remember to laugh more, remember to be flexible and to sort of go with the flow." And then maybe the ten-year-old me is a little bit more uptight or tense, and is saying, "Make sure you're good, make sure you behave, make sure you don't upset anybody." And then I go to the fifteen-year-old me, the next committee member, and maybe this part of me is saying, "No, shake things up, take more risks, be more of an adventurer." And then I go to the next committee member, maybe the twenty-year-old, and that part of me says, "Be more responsible, you can't have that much fun, you've got to take life more seriously." And I can go on and on with more committee members, listening to them one at a time, and giving all of them a chance to have their say, to express their feelings.

And I could go back up the mountain and become the distant watcher for a while, safe and comfortable, but for now I'll stay near the circle and listen as the committee members start to have some conversations with each other. I simply listen and allow the conversations to happen.

And now after letting all the committee members speak and share their feelings about what they feel and what they want, about holding in and letting go, I can use my breathing to return to the mountain, to climb back up to the second watcher perspective, up to my truest self where I can see things with different eyes. From this new point of view, from the mountaintop, looking down with my telescope, with my binoculars or my very clear vision of my everyday life, I can ask myself, after hearing from all the committee members, listening with acceptance, compassion, love: What do I really feel about my relaxing, and going deeper, and letting go, and healing?

Beautiful. I'm learning to listen to myself, what a great present. I could never practice this one too much.

The Committee Meeting is one of the most powerful and versatile trance ideas I can offer you in this book, and you'll see it described several more times in Part II. It can be developed in different settings and used not only with the four ages pictured here, but with any number and kind of self-aspects, such as a mix of feelings on a certain subject, parts of the body, family members, and so on.

• • •

Remember: these are simply ideas to help get you started developing your own trance scripts. Use your personal style and imagery and you'll make your self-hypnosis even more effective. So add your own details, or bend and mold these forms to your own uses and purposes—or dream up some of your own out of your own imagination. Experiment. You give yourself the power to make changes from within. Trust your unconscious mind to come up with the best metaphors and symbol suggestions for you. Your unconscious is only waiting to speak and help you make positive changes.

CHAPTER 7

Ending and Extending
Your Trance

There's more to ending a self-hypnosis session than just opening your eyes and stirring from your chair. In the last few minutes of your trance you can accomplish several important things. You can reorient yourself to the conscious state. You can make suggestions that will extend the effects of your self-hypnosis work beyond the trance session. And you can set up powerful cues that will activate your suggestions in your everyday life.

Take Your Time

Self-hypnosis is a soothing and relaxing experience, so try not to make your last moments hurried. You've achieved a slower and more rhythmical tempo of breathing in your session, and you should try to hold onto this slower pace as you come out of the trance, and even as you return to your busy waking life.

Remember, your breathing is the bridge from your innermost self to your outermost self, from the unconscious to the conscious mind. So when you've finished and feel satisfied with your inner work—when you're ready—just refocus on your breathing, and let yourself slowly retrace your steps back to the surface. Take your time; make it comfortable. Slowly stretching your arms and legs, or maybe your neck, can also help you comfortably reconnect to the outer world. Here's what your trance-ending moments might sound like:

> *I can move around . . . slowly . . . ready to drift into sleep if I want . . . or I can stretch out and awaken from this trance with a refreshed . . . wakeful feeling. Perhaps I'll climb back up some steps . . . or I'll count back up from one to five . . . I might stretch out . . . and feel as if I've awakened from a dream, comfortable . . . refreshed, very naturally, at my own pace . . . 1 . . . 2 . . . feeling more alert . . . 3 . . . my eyes opening . . . 4 . . . 5 . . . alert, awake, and feeling well.*

In the same way, once back in a conscious state, don't be in a hurry to inspect or to analyze your self-hypnosis experience, whatever it's been. The experience of self-hypnosis is in your unconscious mind, and conscious, critical analysis of your thoughts and feelings might well disrupt the ongoing unconscious process. Move right on to some other activity in your waking life, and wait and think about your trance experience a little later, perhaps in a few hours.

Posthypnotic Suggestions and Cues

Although you've now awakened comfortably out of your trance, the work you've just finished can be programmed to go on affecting you positively anytime you desire, well after your self-hypnosis session. This powerful extension of effects is due to what are called posthypnotic suggestions and cues.

What's a posthypnotic suggestion? It's a suggestion given while in trance for an action or response to take place later, in the course of your everyday life.

And what's a posthypnotic cue? It's any action, thought, feeling, word, image, or event that triggers your unconscious mind to act on your suggestion.

By implanting posthypnotic suggestions and cues near the end of your trance session, you can greatly enhance your abilities to change and improve your behavior in your normal, everyday life, not just when you're practicing self-hypnosis. In fact, if it weren't for this remarkable effect, the power of self-hypnosis would be vastly diminished.

For example, suppose your goal in self-hypnosis is to relax and reduce your stress. While in trance you're calm and relaxed, but when faced with a stressful situation at work—maybe a surprise meeting with your boss or a client—you feel your breathing getting quicker, your heart beating faster, and your muscles tensing. You want to calm down, but you don't have time for a self-hypnosis session before the meeting starts.

However, in an earlier session you've given yourself a suggestion to relax at the office, and you've implanted two simple cues to trigger your relaxation response. One cue is to take a few deep breaths, and the other is to uncoil a paper clip. While in self-hypnosis, you've often used deep breathing to relax, so that association is strong; but you've also made a new association of uncoiling a paper clip with unwinding your tense, coiled muscles. Now, at work, with the stress mounting, you take several deep breaths to relax, and you quietly straighten out a paper clip to trigger the release of stress.

Or maybe your goal is losing weight. While in self-hypnosis, you've given yourself the suggestion that whenever you finish a modest and satisfying meal, you'll have a full and content feeling. The cue you've implanted to trigger this full feeling is the act of reaching across the table for a second helping. Now, as with all suggestions, your imagery needs to be as detailed and specific as possible. So you might visualize yourself trying to reach and lift the surprisingly heavy serving dishes, or picture the serving spoons or forks bending under the weight of the extra food.

Here are a few more quick examples:

Grabbing the cold, smooth refrigerator door handle can be a cue for you to avoid in-between-meal snacks.

Pulling down your blankets and fluffing your pillow can be your cue to feel warm, soft, and sleepy.

Seeing the color green (or blue, or your favorite color) anywhere in your daily life can be a cue for feelings of new growth and improved health.

Aligning the strings on your tennis racket can be your cue to concentrate on hitting the next ball on the sweet spot.

The sound of a train rumbling past your house can be a cue for you to take a deep, satisfying breath and relax.

Clearing your throat can be your cue to clear out mental distractions.

Straightening your tie or smoothing your skirt can be a cue for you to straighten or smooth out your personal relations at work.

And, as always, taking a deep, satisfying breath, with a focus on the exhale, can be a cue for you to let go of stress anytime and any place.

Because they're extended influences, posthypnotic suggestions and cues often need to be repeated in several self-hypnosis trance sessions—maybe five or six—before they start to have an effect. Also it's often helpful to give a variety of cues in order to maximize the effect you want. If you give yourself several suggestions and cues, and a few weeks of reinforcement, your unconscious will recognize the association you're making and initiate the desired response.

The Case of Jerry

Jerry, an executive at a top brokerage firm, had a lot of trouble getting to sleep at night. The worries and pressures of his job intensified during the late afternoon and evening until, by 10 P.M., he was too keyed up to sleep. So he stayed up late every night watching TV, and, if he was lucky, got a few hours of restless sleep.

Jerry began learning self-hypnosis to deal with his sleeping problem. While in a trance, he gave himself the suggestion of a new bedtime routine: Each night he would check to make sure the front door was locked, then go directly to bed, read for half an hour, turn out his nightstand light, and grow sleepy.

The first few weeks, he continued regularly repeating his posthypnotic suggestions and cues while in self-hypnosis, and, sure enough, he began to relax more in the evening. His sleeping also gradually improved until night after night he would drift off comfortably soon after going to bed.

At first, Jerry consciously remembered and reviewed his cues—checking the front door lock, reading, turning out the light. But as the weeks went by, he began forgetting about the door lock cue, although he found that he still automatically checked the lock each night. Later on he also forgot about the light being a cue, and yet he would invariably yawn and grow sleepy right after turning the light off at bedtime.

There's nothing mysterious or compulsive about Jerry's behavior. The cues of checking the lock and switching off the light had simply become so firmly implanted in his unconscious—the routine had become so deeply ingrained—that he responded as always, even though he had not consciously reminded himself to do so.

Of course, Jerry could have changed his response had he chosen to. Say that one evening he had finished reading, turned off the light—and the phone rang. He would certainly be free to answer the phone, or to get up to help a friend, or do anything else he needed to. With self-hypnosis, you always have the power to act or not to act, and many studies have shown that you can easily override a cue and change your prearranged response.

Jerry's case is almost textbook because he got everything right. First he had a strong motivation—the need to rest. He also took his time and repeated his suggestions and cues in many sessions over several weeks, which gave his unconscious mind time to respond. His choice of cues was especially effective, since they were numerous and were all closely related to his goal, going to sleep. He might have used other cues, such as brushing his teeth, turning on his electric blanket, or taking off his robe, just as effectively. But less appropriate cues, such as picking up his car keys or tapping his foot, would have had little connection with sleeping, and so would have had a weaker effect. Lastly, his cues were well-designed to be specific, detailed, and positive.

Using these terrific posthypnotic suggestions and cues, Jerry helped himself relax from his high-pressure career and get a good night's sleep. Whatever your personal goals, you can use your imagination in the same way to achieve them.

Cueing Your Next Self-Hypnosis

According to Dr. Milton Erickson, the most important posthypnotic suggestion you can give yourself in trance prepares you to re-enter self-hypnosis whenever and wherever you wish. So, as you close your trance session, just before you count up to consciousness, always try to remind yourself that you can reinstate this pleasant, soothing state quickly and easily, and any time you choose.

For example, you might end your trance with the following suggestion:

I know that I can return to this level of comfort and free-dom any time I wish. Just by taking a few deep, satisfying breaths, I can visualize a stairway leading down from the mountains, or from the coastal bluffs, and return to this level of relaxation.

Each time I practice this form of deep relaxation, it will be easier for me to return. Each time I return, I can become more relaxed, more deeply comfortable, more absorbed and aware. I will find it easier each time.

Now I can return to a refreshed, alert, wakeful state merely by counting from one to five. With each number I count, I become more awake, more alert.

1 . . . 2 . . . 3 . . . 4 . . . 5 . . .

Fully alert, refreshed, and awake. With my eyes wide open.

Of course, deep breathing as a cue is a great old standby, but you can also use any vivid and personal image to initiate a self-hypnotic trance.

The Case of Joan

Joan awoke from her self-hypnotic trance. Her doctor had taught Joan self-hypnosis to help her lose weight—or, more specifically, to help her explore her childhood memories, the better to understand her use of food as a response to emotional turmoil.

The counselor had also taught Joan to visualize an image at the end of her trance session, something colorful and personal she could picture whenever she wanted to re-enter self-hypnosis.

Joan could have used any image, but one stood out for her. As a child, she had once taken a hot air balloon ride at a local carnival. It had been quite a thrill for a little girl, and even as an adult she could vividly remember going up in that big yellow

balloon. So, as she finished her session, Joan gav[e]
suggestion that the next time she wanted to enter th[e]
would close her eyes and visualize a yellow hot air balloon.
she took several deep breaths and counted back from ten
one, she would be in self-hypnosis.

The next evening, when Joan settled in for her self-hypnosis,
she tried it. She leaned back in her comfortable chair in her living room, closed her eyes, and imagined the big yellow balloon.
She took several deep breaths, started counting down from
ten, and before she got to one, she felt herself relaxing and
her hand beginning to get numb—a sure sign she was entering
a self-hypnotic trance.

• • •

It might seem odd to finish this chapter on *ending* your trance
with a description of *entering* another trance. But, then, self-
hypnosis is not a one-time treatment or a quick fix. You need to
repeat your trance work regularly, over the course of several
weeks or months, to begin to see the changes you want. Take all
the time you need—remember, this is time for yourself—and,
like our friend the violinist, practice, practice, practice. You'll
never stop thanking yourself.

CHAPTER 8

ete Trance Script

So far, I've described the three parts of a self-hypnosis session—putting yourself into trance, developing your trance, and coming out of trance. And I've also shown you many bits and pieces of imagery, symbolism, scenarios, and suggestions, some small, others quite extensive. But the whole is always greater than the sum of its parts, and so now I'd like to put everything together and give you a complete script of a trance session. This is only an example, mind you, and as always, you're encouraged to adapt it, or change it entirely, to fit your individual style and your personal goals.

Find a sitting position with your arms resting comfortably and your feet flat on the floor, or maybe with your legs comfortably propped-up and uncrossed. If you wear eyeglasses, remove them, and loosen any constrictive clothing. Adjust your position and become as relaxed as you can. This induction will not use the eye-fixation method, so simply let your eyes grow heavy.

> *To experience even more comfort and relaxation, I'll begin to breathe deeply, maybe I'll take three or four deep, satisfying breaths. As I do this, I'll pay particular attention to the various sensations I experience as I exhale and the air leaves my body.*
>
> *Every breath brings in new air and every exhale gets*

rid of old air. Like a bellows . . . healthy winds flow . . . into me. I can let myself feel as comfortable as I desire with every breath I take in . . . and I can feel even more comfortable with every breath I exhale.

Each outgoing breath gets rid of stress . . . gets rid of worry . . . gets rid of discomfort. I can imagine a tea kettle that is boiling water and see in my mental picture how the steam escapes and relieves the pressure in the kettle. I can let my breath escape in a hissing sound . . . just like the tea kettle . . . releasing unnecessary . . . unneeded pressures and tensions.

I can feel the muscles in my body relaxing. I may notice them first flowing downward from my head . . . through my face . . . through my shoulders . . . down my arms . . . through my chest . . . all the way around my back to my waist. With each breath I exhale, I exhale more tension . . . exhale my troubles all the way out.

As I naturally continue breathing, comfortably and deeply . . . and in rhythm . . . I can begin to picture in my mind a staircase, any kind of staircase, any kind of staircase I choose. Perhaps it's a spiral staircase . . . maybe a staircase from a house I've been in. It might even be a staircase from a movie or television program I've seen. It doesn't matter what shape it is or what it looks like.

I can form an image of it now, in my mind. I can see the banister, the carpeting, and all the details clearly. It may be a staircase from my childhood or one that I completely make up in my mind right now.

The staircase can have any number of steps on it. Perhaps it has ten steps. I can see myself at the top of the stairway. And as I stand there I may be able to notice the smells and the sounds around me. I may hear birds or the sounds of the outdoors, as people move about in their natural daily life . . . just as I am taking time out now, for myself . . . naturally.

And if I hear a car pass by or a plane fly overhead . . . I know that I can imagine all my tension . . . all my stress has been packed into a suitcase or a bag. As the car or plane passes . . . I can imagine myself flinging that bag onto the back of the car, truck, train, or airplane. And as the vehicle passes, and the sounds drift farther away from me . . . I know that my tension and stress are leaving with it.

So in a moment, not yet, but in a moment I'm going to begin moving down the imaginary staircase. I'm going to count each step as I move down. And as I probably already know . . . or maybe even anticipate . . . as I count each number down, I'll become more relaxed . . . more comfortable with each step.

One step for each number that I count. The smaller the number the farther down I go. I may find that there are even more steps than I thought. The farther down I go, the more relaxed and more comfortable I get.

Whether I feel as if my feet are sinking into the carpet, perhaps so deep and so soft, or whether I feel supported by the railing . . . with my hand keeping me steady as I move . . . I know that I'll be more relaxed . . . more comfortable with each step.

I'm going to get ready to begin. Clearly in my mind, right now, I can see or sense the staircase, feel the steps . . . I'm getting ready.

I'm ready now to begin . . . with each step I can feel more relaxed, more comfortable.

10 . . . the first step down the staircase. As the first step in any journey . . . this is often an important one . . . relaxing, getting rid of tension.

9 . . . the second step and I can move as if I'm taking a walk on a comfortable, clear day. The more I walk, the more steps I take, the more I can feel comfortable and distanced from any worries or concerns.

8 . . . on this step, the tension loosens and warmth and coolness can take their place. There are any number of images that may be helpful for me, rivers . . . fields . . . mountains. This staircase can be like any one of them.

7 . . . I may also see many colors. Perhaps the colors of the staircase or of the walls . . . or of the sky or pictures on the walls. The colors may vary from a gray shade to a deep navy . . . but no matter what shade of blue I find myself imagining, I know the color can bring about different things . . . different feelings. The gray can bring about a cool breeze blowing past my body. The brilliant blue can bring the warmth of the sun directly on me.

6 . . . I'm halfway down the staircase. I may see other colors. I may see greens like the grasses outdoors. I may visualize reds or pinks and yellows. Gold, brown, and even black or white can all intermingle . . . mix or stay clearly separate. Whether in a kaleidoscope or individually, I can feel myself using these memories of colors and images to feel as comfortable and as deeply relaxed as I'd like . . . colorful rainbows . . . sails on boats . . . paintings . . . and even balloons. More and more relaxed.

5 . . . and as I descend more, I can feel the relaxation sweep over me, so comfortably, so safely that I know that I can enjoy this experience and return to it again. I know that I can travel wherever I wish. Into the future . . . or into the past . . . with colors or without. I can feel sensations in my fingers . . . I may enjoy feeling a cool wetness . . . perhaps a tingling numbness. I may feel a numbness around my mouth, like a river with cool waters and this is perfectly natural.

4 . . . feeling more and more relaxed.

3 . . . nearing a new level of the stairs. I can feel the warmth in my body and perhaps even coolness. All through me like I'm in a painting or part of the land-scape . . . all around me . . . so personally designed.

2 . . . almost there.

1 . . . I can feel more deeply relaxed. I can take a deep, satisfying breath and feel more calm, more relaxed than maybe ever before. It's as if I've arrived at my peaceful setting.

Perhaps I can even imagine a more peaceful setting now, in my mind. Maybe I'll see some shapes . . . circles . . . triangles . . . or squares. I can even color in the shapes. So I'll color in a circle or a triangle. And whether it's an ancient image of me or a circle that balances me, or whether I can see in my mind's eye the changes in shades and the subtle changes in the shapes or not, it's all there . . . and here . . . and available . . . and healing . . . just by being here now.

I can use my mind's eye to see the changes that I suggest to myself. And as I get ready to do this, I can take a couple of deep . . . satisfying . . . breaths. And I may notice how light or how heavy my body can feel. I might even feel my hands and arms . . . maybe my left . . . or maybe my right, get lighter and feel as if it can float . . . like a leaf . . . safe . . . supported in nature . . . for a while . . . comfort-able . . . secure . . . alive and open . . . in a flow.

I might imagine balloons tied to my arm. Colored bal-loons filled with helium like those I had as a child. The balloons make my arm feel lighter and lighter. My arm may feel as if it wants to float up . . . like a balloon.

Let's see how vividly I can imagine the balloons. I can picture them now. Clearly and colorfully tied to my arm and tugging gently. My arm may even float up a bit off my lap or off the armrest. But whether my arm floats up a little or a lot is not important. I know that the feeling I have right now is of deep comfort and relaxation.

And in just a couple of minutes . . . I'll know that I can make changes in me . . . positive changes that I want to make. I can begin to feel the energy that's been with me all this time . . . beginning to move upward and downward.

I know that social occasions . . . are enjoyable and relaxing diversions. They are also times . . . when I might take better care of myself . . . and remember a very healthy thought . . . that I can avoid overeating. I may be observing others eating . . . I may hear others chewing and see their mouths watering . . . but, as I sip my drink and hear the ice tinkling against the clear glass . . . I am reminded that my body can be lighter than theirs. The clarity and aliveness in my body can be mine . . . by avoiding overeating.

When I open the refrigerator door . . . to find some food to eat between meals . . . instead I may find that I can open a book that I will enjoy. Or I may be able to open the front door and take a brisk walk . . . or perhaps go out in the yard and do some gardening. I may find that taking a walk . . . or a drive . . . can be just as satisfying as eating food. And that closing the door to the refrigerator . . . is just as easy as closing my desire for food. I can close the door and leave behind the food . . . just as I can leave behind my hunger for extra food. I may ask myself . . . what am I really hungry or thirsty for? Companionship? Am I bored and thirsty for excitement?

In a couple of minutes, perhaps sooner than I might expect . . . I may want to finish this experience . . . as I finish many others. And I know that the next time I want to enjoy this same wonderful experience . . . this same relaxation . . . I can re-enter it . . . perhaps more quickly . . .

maybe even easier . . . whenever I take several deep, comfortable breaths.

I might digest new ideas . . . float to new levels . . . and create positive change for life . . . unconsciously and . . . consciously. I might move around . . . slowly . . . ready to drift into sleep if that is my wish . . . or to awaken from this trance with a refreshed . . . wakeful feeling. Perhaps I'll climb back up the stairway, counting from one to ten . . . I'll feel myself going up, and I'll become more alert the closer I get to one.

When I reach the top of the stairs . . . at my own pace . . . I'll awaken feeling refreshed and alert. The closer I get . . . the more awake I'll feel and the more refreshed I'll become.

1 . . . 2 . . . 3 . . . 4 . . . 5 . . . Just like I've taken a long nap, I can begin to awaken and feel well rested, clear, alert, refreshed.

6 . . . 7 . . . 8 . . . 9 . . . 10 . . . A deep refreshing breath, an awakening breath, I feel clear and alert.

The techniques and scripts presented throughout Part I contain many forms of image and suggestion material for gaining relaxation and developing a calm, renewing self-hypnotic trance. After reading this section, you may have a good idea of how to improvise your own inner monologue of suggestions without a written script. That's fine.

You may need to practice several times with any technique before you're completely successful at entering self-hypnosis, or you may find you easily enter a trance the first time you practice. How quickly you develop this skill has no bearing on how effective self-hypnosis will ultimately be for you.

As I've said, be patient with yourself. Change takes time and effort. Set aside some time every day to practice a few minutes of self-hypnosis with a script such as this one. It's not so important how much time you invest—what's important is your intention and motivation during that time. The energy and time you devote to self-change are investments in yourself. You'll be enjoying the dividends for a long time.

Also, the skills you develop in self-hypnosis are lifelong. You need only practice them to keep them sharp and effective. In fact, your skills will grow and expand as you use them and experiment with them.

Now, as you turn to your goal of losing weight and keeping it off, take your self-hypnosis with you and enjoy your new capacity for self-change and better health.

PART II

The Keep It Off Weight-Loss Program

They will often tell me they can't love themselves because they are so fat, or as one girl put it, "too round at the edges." I explain that they are fat because they don't love themselves. When we begin to love and approve of ourselves, it's amazing how weight just disappears from our bodies.

—Louise Hay, *You Can Heal Your Life*

CHAPTER 9

Phase One: Awareness

There's an old saying that goes, "Truth will set you free." When it comes to challenges such as losing weight and keeping it off, I would certainly agree. But I would change the first word to "Awareness." Awareness is what sets you free, it's what liberates you, and so it's the natural starting point in my Keep It Off Weight-Loss Program. No matter if you're enslaved by cravings for food, if you're trapped in a cycle of weight loss and weight gain, or if you're imprisoned by years of repressed feelings, Awareness is the master key that can unlock the door to a healthier, happier life.

What I mean by "Awareness" is taking a good, long look at yourself and your relationship with food. It means looking deep inside yourself at the inner factors—thoughts, feelings, memories—that are the root cause of your weight problem. And it means looking honestly outside yourself at the outer factors— personal relationships, social pressure, eating habits—that also contribute to your overeating.

However, and importantly, "Awareness" in my program is a special kind of looking at yourself and your life. It's observation without judgment or criticism, it's watching what happens without trying to change what happens, it's attention without tension. And this is where self-hypnosis plays a vital role, because, as you learned in Part I, self-hypnosis brings you quickly and effectively to this state of calm, absorbed awareness, detached and yet interested, distanced and yet curious. In practical terms, "Awareness" means seeing yourself from the Second Watcher perspective that I described in Chapter 6—sitting in the back row of a theater and watching yourself watch the movie of your life.

By using self-hypnosis for awareness, you can explore your weight problem inside and out. You can begin to identify the ways you use food to relieve stress, to meet emotional needs, or to avoid uncomfortable feelings. You can also start to take notice of the personal and social situations that stimulate overeating. And you can start to recognize ways other than eating to help you cope with life.

Remember food is not your problem; it is, for now, your best solution to your problems. But not for long. With self-hypnosis, you can enter a relaxed state of watchfulness, of effortless awareness of all sides of your weight problem, which can free you to find other more positive and permanent solutions.

What Do You Weigh Inside?

Since weight loss (or weight gain, for that matter) happens from the inside out, the first thing you need to become aware of is how much you weigh inside. Yes, that's right, not your outer, physical weight, but your inner, emotional weight.

Let me explain what I mean. We all carry around within us positive and negative life experiences, imprinted on us from our childhood to the present moment, and the nature of these experiences determines our emotional weight. Positive, healthy experiences create in us a sense of lightness and joyfulness; negative, hurtful experiences create a sense of heaviness and depression.

Now, because our negative experiences usually involve an inner conflict or struggle, we don't often deal openly and honestly with the emotions they produce (sadness, fear, loneliness, anger, guilt, etc.). Rather than accepting, expressing, and resolving these difficult feelings, we bury them inside our bodies, where they grow strong and take their revenge through all sorts of excessive behaviors, including overeating.

In this case, when we stuff ourselves with negative emotions, our emotional weight balloons. And the trouble is that when our emotional weight soars, our body weight usually does the same. My years of working with overweight people, both in my private practice and at Kaiser Permanente, have proven to me that the heavier you feel emotionally or psychologically, the more likely you are to be heavy physically.

How much do you weigh emotionally? How many heavy thoughts and feelings have you swallowed and stored inside your body? Begin to find some answers by taking the following quiz. Complete all sixteen statements by circling the "a" or "b" responses. Be as honest as you can be. Don't repress, judge, or criticize your responses. There are no right or wrong answers.

The Oceana Quiz for Emotional Weight

1. Memories of my mother are
    a. distressing and unhappy much of the time
    b. peaceful and happy much of the time

2. My parents' relationship was often
    a. troubled and strained
    b. loving and mutually respectful

3. When I'm upset about something, I'm most likely to
    a. keep it to myself
    b. talk it out with someone

4. When I think of my father, I usually feel
    a. a sense of distance and coolness
    b. a sense of closeness and warmth

5. When dealing with "authority figures" I most often feel
   a. intimidated
   b. self-confident

6. My mother showed me affection
   a. with difficulty and only occasionally
   b. naturally and quite often

7. As a child, I
   a. felt I had to hide my feelings
   b. felt free to share my feelings

8. Sex education was taught to me in
   a. unwelcome circumstances that confused me
   b. an appropriate way at the right time

9. In my relationship with myself I tend to be
   a. hard on myself
   b. in support of myself

10. In my family, alcohol was
   a. abused and caused problems
   b. used appropriately for special occasions

11. My father played with me
   a. rarely and with difficulty
   b. regularly and easily

12. Love is something I feel
   a. distrustful of
   b. comfortable with

13. My home life as a child was
   a. often changing and inconsistent
   b. stable and consistent

14. My family
   a. had trouble showing affection
   b. was warm and loving

15. My body usually feels
    a. stressed and uncomfortable
    b. relaxed and comfortable

16. If I made a mistake, my parents
    a. criticized me
    b. supported me

Scoring

The number of your "a" responses is a good indicator of how much emotional weight you're carrying around inside in the form of repressed feelings. Count up your "a" responses and locate yourself on the following scale of emotional weight.

1 to 4 "a" Responses: Light Emotional Weight

Life has its light, comfortable moments, just as your physical weight is usually pretty comfortable—although you could always take off a few pounds. But for you, this isn't enough. You're determined to do better in life, and you want to become your healthiest weight.

If your emotional weight score places you in this category, your repressed feelings get you down sometimes but they're usually manageable. You need to stop focusing on what's wrong with you and learn to simply accept yourself and appreciate what's right about you. Remember, you are *already* that which you can become. All you need are the right skills to help you tap into your creativity and find new answers to old problems.

5 to 8 "a" Responses: Heavy Emotional Weight

Life has its ups and downs, and your physical weight may also fluctuate. Some things in your life are okay but many things are not, and you often find yourself feeling blue—sometimes even gripped by fear and worry. You've traveled a long road to reach this point, but happiness still eludes you. As soon as you take care of one thing, another turns up.

If your emotional weight score places you in this category, you need to learn to see life's twists and turns through new eyes. The skills that will help you the most are those that enhance your emotional flexibility. Remember, you're not *just* your experiences, or your moods, or your feelings. You already know how to observe and listen to these things and your self . . . and you'll be learning more about how to integrate your self-hypnosis/self-care skills into your daily life.

9 to 12 "a" Responses: Severe Emotional Weight

Life seems a burden much of the time, something you have to carry around like your excess weight. You're more than likely struggling with feeling overweight and stressed out. You wish you had time to learn to relax and be well. Relaxing sounds like a good idea, but right now you're too busy. You try to overcome adversity, to gain insight and direction. You often succeed, but it's so much effort and stress. You wish there was some way to lighten the load.

If your emotional weight score places you in this category, you're fighting with yourself—and you're losing the battle because you're repressing your feelings. You need to get the past behind you, and start living more in the present, with one foot in the present, and one foot into the future. Remember, happiness is not just out of your reach. Happiness is always *within* you, when you're taking the best care of yourself possible. Your relationship with yourself is as important as all the others that really matter to you, and it affects all the others.

13 to 16 "a" Responses: Dangerous Emotional Weight

Life for you is a challenging trial. You spend a great deal of time in the grip of unhappy thoughts and stressful feelings. You experience many physical discomforts—perhaps a nervous stomach, body aches, or other nagging illnesses. Very likely weight has been a serious issue at some time in your life. Maybe a good deal too much weight. And maybe for most of your life.

If you're in this category, your repressed feelings are working against you. You need to learn to let these feelings go by giving them a voice of their own. Remember, the holding in of tension is *dis*-ease and the expression of feelings is *heal*-thy. Accept and let go—one feeling at a time. For you, overeating and being overweight have been coping skills. They're the best way you've figured out to take care of yourself . . . up until now. They've worked well for you—good job—but your life can be a lot better now. Ready?

So, having found that you need to let go of some emotional weight, what do you do now? The answer is, don't do anything. Don't try to lose weight, inner or outer. Just become more aware.

The Compassion Response

First, however, you may be wondering if all of this inner work—becoming aware of your buried feelings, troubled relationships, difficult memories, or anything else you've avoided dealing with—will make you feel worse before you feel better. Don't worry.

The amazing thing about awareness through self-hypnosis is that it feels so right, it feels so good. No matter how difficult the feelings or memories you explore in self-hypnosis, when you become more fully aware of them a deeper peace prevails. Instead of hurting as you bring them to light, you feel calm and relaxed, open-minded and welcoming. Very likely you'll also feel a greater understanding of how absurd life can be, and you might even laugh a little at how seriously you've been taking things.

This generosity of mind and spirit is so characteristic of self-hypnosis that I'm tempted to call it a "compassion response." You see, when you've relaxed your critical, ambitious, ego-driven conscious mind, you're able to access your more loving and creative unconscious mind—and you immediately begin to see yourself and others through new eyes of compassion and tolerance. So it doesn't matter what weight-related problems, dilemmas, or conflicts you're becoming aware of in your self-hypnosis. When you enter trance, your natural response will be to feel relaxed, compassionate, caring, and friendly toward yourself, and toward all of the other people in your life, past and present.

Explore the Starting Point

Here is a self-hypnosis awareness trance to help you dig down to the root feelings and memories that might be at the bottom of your weight problem.

Before entering self-hypnosis, set your goal in writing. For example, write down for yourself, "I want to better understand why I began to overeat." The goal should be specific and open to all possibilities.

Second, be aware that you're dealing with many issues that are difficult to express. Be aware of the challenge; don't pretend with yourself. Still, be open to exploring issues that may come up for you during the trance. Encouraging your own openness to hidden material may lead you to find options that can help you break down conscious resistance to change.

Third, try to notice when you feel yourself closing in on an important issue. Pause for a moment and review it privately in your own mind. Talk to yourself (out loud or silently), and write down any words and ideas that can help you understand more about any issues that seem important.

And fourth, make this work of self-awareness a priority. Make a commitment to plan a schedule for practicing—once a day, twice a day, or whatever time you can devote. You decide how often and how long you can spend practicing, but respect your desire to make a significant change in your life.

So, after you've taken several deep breaths, relaxed, and walked down your stairway into a comfortable trance . . .

You might remember a happy and healthy time in your life when excess weight was not an issue. Let your unconscious mind take you back to that time before you began overeating. Go over an entire day if you can, from getting up in the morning to going to bed at night. Pay particular attention to your meals. Remember as many details as possible.

Next, try to remember an unhappy and unhealthy time when gaining weight became an issue in your life. Go over the situation step by step; discover the first time you experienced the overeating problem. Be honest about your feelings, and trust your unconscious to know what's important and what's not important. Let your unconscious be your guide. If your mind drifts, go with it; mental side trips can be more valuable than you think.

You may ask yourself, is there some past event responsible for your overeating, being overweight or being unsatisfied? Was it before you were twenty years old? Was it before you were ten years old? Was it before you were five years old?

Try to recall what was happening at the time. Try to remember details. When you know what it was, you'll feel more relaxed and you'll be able to describe it to yourself or write it down.

You may ask yourself, is it all right to tell yourself about it?

You may ask yourself, is there an earlier experience that might have set the stage or made you vulnerable to overeating, being overweight, or being unsatisfied?

You may ask yourself, is there anything else you need to know before you can feel free of the extra weight?

You may ask yourself, now that you know this, can you be well?

You'll probably have to work with this trance for several self-hypnosis sessions before you begin to see results. Be patient and listen to your unconscious mind. When it's ready, it will tell you all you need to know about when to expect a change in your weight.

What Are the Advantages of Being Overweight?

As you become more aware of the deep-seated emotional reasons for being overweight, you also need to ask yourself if you can think of any reasons why you might want to *remain* overweight. This might seem like a strange idea—that you'll resist losing weight, even as you're committed to losing weight. But search yourself, deeply, and you might very well find that you have powerful unconscious reasons for wanting to hold on to your weight and keep life just as it is.

Ask yourself the difficult question: What are the advantages of staying overweight? Be honest with yourself—there could be some well-hidden secrets involved here. Then write a list of what you come up with. For example:

1. Less is expected of a fat person
2. Weight can be a protective shield
3. Being fat reduces sexual threat
4. No one bothers a big person
5. Being heavy gains you sympathy
6. Losing weight is threatening to others

Let's look at two related points: (2) "protective shield" and (3) "reduces sexual threat." How does being overweight protect you sexually?

Well, suppose for some reason you're shy or insecure, and you fear dating. By making sure you stay overweight, you believe that you can avoid being seen as physically attractive or appealing, and that therefore you'll be left alone. Avoiding such apparently flattering notice might seem odd on the face of it. But underneath you might find it less threatening to hide inside your weight and not put yourself into a more intimate and sexually frightening situation.

Such unconscious reasons are very real for many people, and are worth exploring as you begin learning how to lose weight. If you feel something blocking your progress and you can't get at it on your own, you may wish to seek assistance from a trained hypnotherapist. There are times when a serious early trauma such as molestation, physical injury, or emotional abuse are at the bottom of your unconscious resistance, and these cases can best be helped by professional counseling. (Referrals in your area can be obtained from your doctor, counselor, family member, or friend—anyone you know who has successfully worked with self-hypnosis or medical hypnosis. Or you can contact me personally at www.selfhypnosisisweightloss.com.)

Beware of False Motivation

There are other inner resistances to investigate. Sometimes people who say they want to break a habit—such as overeating— really don't want to break the habit at all. They're only saying they do, perhaps because of family pressure or social expectation. So they enter a program to lose weight, but then they sabotage themselves to make sure they fail. Losing weight is a challenge, and keeping it off is an even greater challenge. To succeed, you need to make a 100 percent commitment, and it has to be a completely self-motivated decision.

How do you know if you really want to lose weight? Give the following awareness exercise some honest thought.

Ask yourself about why you want to lose weight:

1. What are you saying to yourself—inside—about this issue?
2. Are you trying to lose weight because you *should*?
3. Secretly do you already know this won't work?
4. Are you trying to please someone else?
5. Are you trying to prove something?

Now, close your eyes, take a deep breath, and ask yourself, what will you say to yourself if you succeed?

Then ask yourself, what will you say to yourself if you fail?

Breathe through Your Cravings

Breathing is an excellent mirror of your inner life, and becoming aware of your breathing is a quick way to tell how you're dealing with your feelings.

Observe your breathing over a day or two. If it's generally tight and shallow, or if you're exhaling a little and inhaling a lot, then you're holding onto your feelings, a sure sign that you're uncomfortable or unsatisfied with yourself or your life. And of course this spills over into your eating. If you're not satisfied with yourself somehow, or if you need something to make you feel better, you'll try to satisfy yourself with food. It's that simple. You know this doesn't work, not for very long anyway, but you feel as though you have to do something.

Once your breathing is full and deep, however, you're in an open, expressive flow, and your inner heaviness immediately starts to lift. This happens with any of the feelings you've repressed—anger, fear, sadness, loneliness—and even with any bad moods, negative thoughts, or cravings for food. Anything and everything. Just change your breathing from short and shallow to deep and satisfying, and the uptight feeling, mood, or mind set will soon disappear.

Try this awareness exercise whenever you feel the urge to eat:

Don't try to stop overeating. Do only one thing. . . . Breathe.

Before you grab that food, close your eyes and breathe deeply for five minutes. Inhale deeply, exhale deeply. Push the exhale, throw out all the air.

Let go . . . let go . . . *let go.* Breathe into relaxation. Breathe into awareness. Give yourself a loving feeling through breathing and awareness.

Drink a glass of cleansing, refreshing water. Feel better and feel more alive.

You know, with more awareness, you can breathe your way through anything. So the next time you have a craving or just need something to feel better (and food has worked in the past), all you need to do is notice your breathing. Observe your inhale and exhale, particularly your inhale. Accept your breathing as it is, focus on the cycle, pause for a moment at the turning points, and you'll be in a beautiful, relaxed, healthy, comfortable state, and your mood, your thought, your craving will have gotten so small it may have completely disappeared.

Learn Your Eating Triggers

Overeating is triggered by stressful situations in your life, situations that involve external events, other people, issues, memories, and inner turmoil. For instance, you might find that you suddenly want to eat when you're talking to your mother on the phone, or when you're feeling lonely, or when you're thinking about your boss or your finances. By becoming more aware of your triggers, you can free yourself from their control over you.

When you find yourself getting upset, anxious, or in conflict, and then a voice inside says, "I have to eat something," see if this exercise helps:

When you find yourself feeling stressed or upset with yourself, another person, or an issue, set aside one hour to let yourself worry, feel bad, sad, mad, or even worse. Every day at the same time. No judgment or self-criticism. Just watch your feelings, witness them, like being at a movie.

After three days, pick a different hour. This time, be aware of accepting your feelings and believing in yourself. Focus on trusting yourself, loving yourself, and going with the stress. Be aware that all problems enter and exit, like clouds floating across the sky.

Remember, you can stress out as much as you like during your hour the first three days. You're learning to go with it—like following a river. No need to push it—it won't help. No need to fight it—that won't help either. Just enjoy your awareness and the acceptance that flows with it.

The Overeating Response

At the heart of your triggering event, issue, relationship (whatever it is) there is a feeling, which tickles a thought for food, which develops into a desire, which takes on a life of its own and becomes an action. This is the arc of your overeating response: Feeling leads to thought, leads to desire, leads to action.

It helps to know about this path your overeating travels, so that you can gauge how fully your trigger controls you. Here are four stages of awareness that you're in the grip of your overeating response.

1. Post-Awareness. After the act, when it's too late: "I wasn't hungry. I ate because I was upset."
2. During-Awareness. While you're in the act: "I'm eating even though I'm not hungry, and I see I'm upset."

3. Pre-Awareness. Before the act, when a thought is not yet fully planted: "I can tell I'm upset and my impulse is to grab some chocolate."
4. Full-Awareness: watching the whole process as a feeling turns into action. "I know I'm upset. I'll watch myself. I'll be more aware and not make the usual escape to food."

By becoming aware of where you are with your trigger, you have a better chance of catching the feeling before it becomes a thought, or a desire, or an action. Don't try to stop or change your triggers. Use awareness instead.

The Committee Meeting, Part 1

Allowing yourself to be aware of all your emotions and triggers is an important step in getting free of them. But it's also freeing to become aware of how your conscious mind gets in your way. For most of us, the mind is often a jumble of different, even conflicting thoughts and feelings, changing every moment. One moment we're filled with doubt about ever being able to lose weight, and the next moment we're full of belief— then wait a moment and we're doubtful again. One moment we're committed to being healthy and happy, another moment we want to escape. One moment we're loving towards our self and others, then the wheel turns and we're full of anger and hate.

It's like an unruly committee meeting, attended by various parts of yourself to discuss your weight loss goals. Sitting around the conference table are all the usual committee members: your Anger, Fear, Sadness, Will Power, Guilt, your Inner Child, your Inner Parent, your Ideal Self. You might also have given Hope a committee seat, or Doubt, or Indulgence, or the Trim You, or the Fat You. There might be only three or four parts of you at the meeting, or many more.

For a moment Will Power takes the floor, and in that moment you decide not to eat after six P.M. Hope seconds the motion. But then Indulgence stands up and, ignoring Will Power, urges you to give yourself a treat. So one moment you're determined to follow your schedule, the next moment you're searching through the pantry. And you may be surprised—just a minute ago you had decided to eat less and the decision seemed so 100-percent trustworthy. And now it's all gone, gone down the drain, nothing left of it, and you're perfectly willing to overeat again. Then Guilt speaks up and tortures you, and you'll feel stressed and in the next moment you'll feel like a failure.

Be assured that this will go on and on. The mind is always changing. It's a committee meeting of minds. And most people live and die stuck in committee.

Only one thing in you is steady and constant and unchanging in this mental free-for-all. This is your "eye" (or authentic "I") at the center of the storm: The Second Watcher. The Second Watcher is the master of awareness, and can serve as a committee chairperson who sits quietly in the corner and listens and observes the various competing roles and voices in your head.

Enter a Committee Meeting self-hypnosis trance chaired by the Second Watcher. (See Chapter 6 for trance script ideas.) Let the Second Watcher be aware of all the things you're thinking and feeling, and ask, "What part of me is this coming from? Whose voice is it?" Take some time and allow this experience to happen. Go around the room and observe each part of you, listen to each statement, without judgment or criticism. This is a powerful trance that you can use over and over again, each time learning something more about what thoughts, feelings, and memories are influencing you.

Pause Buttons

Another way of looking at the conscious mind is as a tape player that never stops playing your social programming tapes—those prerecorded speeches, thoughts, and opinions about food, calories, how you look, social expectations, "shoulds and shouldn'ts," what other people are thinking of you, on and on. It's a nuisance. It doesn't help you; it doesn't motivate you. In fact, it tends to make you feel worse, eat more, and stay stuck in a rut, playing the same old "song" over and over.

Fortunately, the mind/tape player has a pause button you can push to quiet yourself, relax, stop the panic, let go of fear and self-criticism, and refocus on your goals. If you can find this pause button, you can become more aware of your true, authentic self, and so make clear, positive, healthy decisions about your life, your weight-loss goals, and your relationships.

Naturally, the technique is simple. You can learn this in one minute and it will help you for the rest of your life. You can do this now, a few times during the day, before or during meal times, or whenever you want to get through a food craving, let go, feel strong, relaxed, and even able to giggle at yourself.

First, rate how noisy, active, and over-thinking your mind is on a scale of one to ten, with one being a quiet mind and ten being a busy mind. Most people report something seven or above.

Okay, now inhale a full breath . . . and then exhale and hum at the same time.

Yes, hum. You can hum with your eyes open or closed, although closing your eyes will give you a better and faster effect.

Make sure you hum louder than you've been thinking. Hum as loud as you would sing a song in the shower. You can try different tones and volumes until you find the one that's sweetest to your ears. A tone that feels like you, high-pitched, moderate, or deep, and that comes right from your center.

When you exhale, hum all the way to the end of your breath. Feel your own vibration. The longer you can hum, the faster you will find the pause button, quiet your mind, and feel more self-control.

Do this for about a minute, or for about twenty breaths, where you inhale big and hum on the exhale until the end of your breath.

After twenty breaths, use the same scale from one to ten and note what number now best represents how quiet or busy your mind is. Most people report a one, two, or three.

So, in one minute, you have quieted your mind by humming, and you feel centered, relaxed, and free. This is huge in helping you lose weight and keep it off. Do this humming whenever you get stressed, can't quiet your mind, or feel an overpowering urge to eat.

Speak Your Inner Language

Another great pause button for a quiet mind is the universal and special language called Gibberish. You've spoken it before, though maybe not since you were a baby. At that time, in diapers, before you learned the outer language of your culture, you spoke your own inner language. It was an effortless flow of Gibberish, and it calmed you, delighted you, helped you feel good, made you laugh, and quieted your mind.

Na ka ra la sho pa noo noo la tea da. That is Gibberish. Say this out loud: Ma la too too in so cha cha by the bo bo at win zo zo. If that was fun, do it again. This may sound silly, but by speaking Gibberish you're learning to express yourself again from your center, and it will help you clear your mind, have fun, get out of your own way, find the pause button, let go of stress, laugh at yourself, and refocus on losing weight and keeping it off—all at the same time.

Make up your own Gibberish, or keep repeating the sentences above, for one to two minutes. Watch what happens. You'll have found another pause button in your mind. This is like clearing out the cobwebs. You'll feel clearer as a result of being creative, playful, funny, and relaxed.

Speak Gibberish aloud to yourself for one or two minutes every day. The more you have fun with it, the more you'll feel relaxed and focused on your weight loss goals. Remember: Quiet mind, more peaceful, more aware, more honest.

Tension Food *vs.* Relaxation Food

There are two types of food. One is tension food and it's very tempting, very appealing to your conscious mind. You go into a restaurant and you smell something rich and wonderful coming from the kitchen, or you see someone at the next table with a great looking dinner, or someone brings goodies to work. You see this food, you become interested in it, and you eat it. Or maybe you were doing something else, not thinking of food at all, and suddenly junk food pops into your mind. This is all mind-game food. You were not thinking about it, but there it is, and suddenly you want it. It was not your intention, or your desire, but your hunger was stimulated.

The other kind of food is relaxation food—food that makes you relax. This is food that your body desires because it's nourishing and nurturing for health, wellness, normal weight, and happiness. Your body knows and will ask for what it needs. Studies have shown that if small children are left alone with food, they will eat what is best for their bodies. For example, if a child has a cold, and there is an orange, the child will choose the orange. Even if other foods are available, the child will make the healthy choice.

Now, you can eat tension food but it will not be satisfying, at least not for very long, because it was not your real desire. No matter how much you eat of it, you won't feel satisfied, because your body doesn't need it, and didn't really want it in the first place. You might feel full, but you won't feel satisfied. What's worse, obsession with food comes out of this kind of dissatisfaction. It's true satisfaction you're looking for to lose weight and keep it off.

Relaxation food is deeply satisfying in this way because your desire for it comes from a place inside yourself—your unconscious mind—an intimate place of self-care that you can trust to tell you what you really need. You can eat as much relaxation food as you want and you'll feel right, you'll feel relaxed, and you'll eat like a normal person, because it will satisfy your body.

To discover your favorite relaxation foods, practice this awareness exercise.

Every day, before you eat any food, maybe just before each meal, close your eyes, take a few deep breaths, and ask yourself what you want, what your true desire is. Don't think about what's available in your pantry or in your refrigerator, just pay attention to what your body wants. It might be anything. You haven't seen or smelled any food. You're simply listening to your own feelings, to what your body needs, to what you feel like inside.

Then go and find that food and eat it. Eat as much of it as you wish, but stick with that food. Eat slowly. Eat deliberately. Focus on your body as you swallow. You'll stop eating when you're full. Your body will know when it's satisfied.

Most people never listen to their inner desire for food. Maybe they've forgotten how to consult their body, or maybe they've never been taught how to listen to their inner voice. And so they eat only tension food, and they're dissatisfied, and this can make them obsessed with food, and then they're driven to overeat. That's how the mind game works.

But if you listen to your body and eat relaxation food, the cravings for tension food will be gone. Your answers are in your body. Just eat your relaxing food for a few days, and you'll see that the tension foods will lose their appeal.

Discover the Joy of Eating

There's a difference between eating food and filling yourself with food. And this difference is awareness. If you're aware as you eat, then you're fully experiencing your meal; if you aren't aware, then you're simply indulging your appetite. The experience of eating is beautiful and natural and joyous; indulgent eating is ugly and mechanical and indifferent.

When you're aware of your eating, you naturally enjoy your food, and so you eat only as much as you need. On the other hand, when you're just stuffing food into your body, you don't enjoy it—you can't enjoy it, because you're not *there* to enjoy it. Physically you're eating, but mentally and emotionally you're somewhere else, maybe a million miles away. And so, robot-like, you keep eating until your mealtime is over, or until your plate is clean, or until you finish thinking about whatever it is you're thinking about.

But when you experience your food, when you're totally present and aware, you truly enjoy it. And if you truly enjoy your food, you can't keep mindlessly overeating, or eating un-healthy, empty food. If you experience and enjoy your food totally, your weight loss and weight maintenance will occur naturally.

Self-hypnosis can help you gain more awareness and enjoyment in your eating. Breathe, relax, and get yourself comfortably into trance . . .

> *Imagine you're eating a meal, anything you want. Be as vivid as you can in your imagery, sights, sounds, smells, textures. Then imagine a camera on your shoulder, or just to your side, watching and filming you as you eat. Be that watcher, be that camera. Watch yourself, observe yourself. Notice your mood, your attitude, how tense or relaxed you are. Observe your breathing, shallow or deep. Watch how you hold your knife and fork. Smell the food. Watch the food as it goes into your mouth. How do you chew? Do you really taste? Do you notice the flavors? Watch the food as it goes into your stomach. Is your stomach happy to receive it?*

The amazing thing is that just by becoming more aware of how you eat, your eating will change by itself. Will power doesn't work; you already know that. Only through effortless awareness, not trying to change a thing, can you free yourself to find a lighter and more joyous way of eating.

The Fine Art of Eating

When you get finer and finer in your awareness, you can actually make eating an artistic experience. As I've said, most of us shovel our food in, chew it a bit, swallow quickly, and hardly even taste it. Some of us eat while thinking about a boyfriend, a girlfriend, a job, money, anything but the food. Some of us eat to get it over with because we're in a hurry to do something else. Some of us chat with our friends, watch TV, read the paper, smoke, totally unaware of what we're tasting and eating.

But eating doesn't have to be that way. You can learn the fine art of eating.

This means eating and doing nothing else—the act of eating becomes 100 percent of your focus. No concerns or distractions come between you, your awareness, and your experience of food. You forget about everything else. You take your time. You become sensual, allowing the tastes, smells and textures to be more intense. You taste every bite, inhale all of the aromas, enjoy the colors, and feel the textures. You savor your food. You relax while you eat. You make each meal a simple, direct, and exquisite experience. A work of art.

The next time you eat something try this awareness exercise:

Touch, smell, and taste your food as if you were eating it for the first time. Raise it to your nose and smell the fragrances. Look at your food closely. What shape is it? How many shades of color does it have? Put it in your mouth—but don't chew it yet. Just move it around in your mouth. Can you notice different flavors in different parts of your mouth? Now chew it and listen. What can you hear? Crackling, swishing, crunching? Are the sounds coming from the food or from inside you? What texture does it have? Grainy, spongy, crisp? How hot or cold is it? What aftertaste does it leave?

Tune into your senses, and you'll stop eating when your food stops tasting good. You'll forget cleaning your plate. You'll forget three meals a day. You'll be aware of what your body tells you, and stop when you're no longer hungry.

So, let your awareness of tasting and eating become an artistic experience. Let yourself rediscover the sensual, aesthetic beauty of eating, and you'll cherish your food as well as your body.

Planting the Seeds of Commitment

As I mentioned earlier, meeting the challenge of losing weight and keeping it off requires you to be 100 percent committed to your goal. To make this kind of total commitment, you need to have both your everyday conscious mind (around 10 percent of your awareness) and your deeper unconscious mind (the other 90 percent) united in their focus. Presumably (since you're reading this book), you've made a conscious decision to deal with your weight problem. But you also need your unconscious to be with you all the way.

The following awareness exercise and self-hypnotic trance will help make sure your unconscious mind has heard the signal loud and clear:

When you wake in the morning, be aware of your determination to lose weight and keep it off. Lie still in your warm, half-conscious state, and for five minutes before you get up be aware of your commitment to yourself. Visualize yourself making healthy choices, handling difficult situations beautifully, with self-confidence and self-esteem, and feeling optimistic about your whole day's success with your goal.

Then at night when you go to bed, be aware of your determination to lose weight and keep it off. When you lie down in bed, breathe deeply and review your day, focusing on what was right about your eating, your physical activities, your choices, attitude, awareness, and successes. As you relax and become drowsy, be aware of your goal for five minutes and repeat it to yourself in thought as you go to sleep.

Now here's a way to plant your seeds of success even deeper within. Relax your body and descend into trance as you take several deep, satisfying breaths. When you're ready . . .

On the last breath, exhale completely and then stop your-
self from inhaling for as long as you can. Be aware that in
a matter of moments every pore of your body and millions
of cells will be hungry for air. The longer you hold your
breath, the deeper the longing for breath is going to spread
into your unconscious mind. The longer you hold your
breath, the more the innermost part of your being is going
to ask for air. And if you hold it to the last moment, your
whole being will demand air. It might even feel like a
matter of life and death.

In that moment, when you reach the state where your
whole being is starving for air, repeat to yourself, "I will
lose weight and keep it off. I am aware of my commitment
to my health and happiness." In this state, let your mind
repeat these thoughts, "I will lose weight and keep it off. I
am aware of my commitment to my health and happi-
ness." Your body will ask for air and your mind will repeat
these thoughts, "I will lose weight and keep it off. I am
aware of my commitment to my health and happiness."
The stronger the demand for air, the deeper your aware-
ness and commitment will enter inside. And if all of you
is struggling for air and you're repeating these sentences,
then the strength of your awareness and commitment will
increase many times over.

Do this every day. Add it into your wake up or bedtime routine. Or do it during your day: Exhale five times, wait as long as
possible to inhale, and repeat your ideas inside five times. And
in a matter of two or three days, you'll observe a significant
change. Of course, if you have any heart problems, or any other
health or breathing problem, don't do it strenuously. Do it as
gently as possible and don't make yourself uncomfortable.

The Third Eye

You must have heard about the third eye. You have two regular eyes and they're for seeing outward. But you also have a third eye, right in between your eyebrows, and it's for seeing inward. Of course, there is no third eye physically in your forehead; it's a metaphor for learning how to see inward with your self-hypnosis techniques. By practicing the exercises and trance ideas in this chapter, you're training your third eye to look inward, and in the process you're becoming more aware, more relaxed, with less tension in the mind, with fewer expectations or agendas. You're seeing yourself from the Second Watcher perspective, and this effortless, self-accepting, and self-nurturing Awareness is the foundation for feeling lighter about yourself. Freedom is the goal and Awareness is the master key for self-understanding, self-care, and self-hypnosis.

As you now know, change happens first on the inside and then on the outside. So look inward and see things with a different eye—your third eye. You'll become aware that the power to lose weight and keep it off is within you. And you'll become aware that it's been there all along.

CHAPTER 10

Phase Two: Acceptance

In my study of meditation, I came across an intriguing saying: "Acceptance is Transcendence." Milton Erickson and I had many conversations about how perfectly this saying captured something essential in his teachings. Basic to the Ericksonian method is the notion that whatever personal problem you have in life, whatever barrier is blocking your progress, the way you get past it, the way you overcome it, is not by fighting *against* the problem, not by storming the barrier, but by accepting yourself just as you are.

Now, Dr. Erickson certainly knew the healing power of Awareness—he invented a number of self-observation or self-awareness techniques. But he also understood that Awareness by itself wasn't enough to change firmly entrenched and stoutly defended habits such as overeating. He taught his students and his patients that accepting yourself, even loving yourself—totally and unconditionally—was an essential second step in the process of breaking free. Awareness might be the master key to unlocking the door to change, but Acceptance is the positive action of opening the door and stepping into the daylight and fresh air.

I want to emphasize that Acceptance is a "positive action," because it's easy to think "accepting" means submitting or resigning yourself to a problem—means giving in, maybe even giving up. In fact the opposite is true. Acceptance is pro-active,

).

..., it creates momentum, it opens doors. ...d I don't use the word "miracle" very ...:ept yourself as you are, positive changes

...d diet programs don't understand about ... management, and it's why they have a ... long as you're judging yourself, or judging your body, or juuging the way you eat or the way you look; as long as you're critical of yourself, or you're putting yourself down for being overweight; as long as you make self-acceptance conditional, saying, "Well, okay, I'll accept myself *after* I lose twenty pounds," you're not going to have any success losing weight or keeping it off. It's almost impossible. None of that works.

However, when you accept yourself unconditionally, when you accept your body, when you accept your eating habits, when you accept that food has been your way of dealing with problems, when you accept that food is how your family taught you to cope, when you accept that you don't want to exercise, when you accept that you don't want to change the way you eat—when you accept all your weight issues, all your concerns, all the things that bother you the most about being heavy, then you immediately start to make a change for the better.

And not just a change in your ability to lose weight and keep it off. You'll also begin to feel better about yourself, to form healthier habits, to improve your relationships with others, and to take better care of yourself than perhaps you've ever done in your life.

The Breath of Life

A good place to start learning about accepting yourself is with your breathing. Remember, your breath is your life, and when you accept your breathing as it is, you naturally begin to accept yourself as you are.

The following self-hypnotic trance can help you explore the connection between your breathing and your self-acceptance. As you're relaxing and falling into trance . . .

Focus on your breathing, on the rise and fall of each breath. Accept your breathing as it is. Recognize that word, "accept." Accept your breathing as it is. Nose or mouth, it really doesn't matter. Deep or light, it really doesn't matter. Throat or belly, it really doesn't matter. Deep or shallow, it really doesn't matter. Rough or smooth, it really doesn't matter. Tense with lots of thoughts or calm with just one, it really doesn't matter. Simply accept your breathing as it is. Just focus on the rise and fall of each breath and accept your breathing as it is.

Now put your awareness on the moment when your inhale turns into an exhale . . . and then again when your exhale turns into an inhale. There's a turning point in every breath you'll ever take, have ever taken, and they last about a millisecond. That's right. See if you can accept these turning points without trying to change them. Notice when they come . . . how long they last . . . and when they begin to turn. Accept them as they are, these moments when your inhale turns into an exhale and then again when your exhale turns into an inhale.

And you might see that there's the tiniest pause in the middle of each turning point, a split-second moment of silence poised between the inhale and the exhale. In observing that silent pause there's beauty, that's right, and something very grand and simple at the same time. It's what it feels like to accept yourself as you are.

The Committee Meeting, Part 2

Perhaps the biggest obstacle to effective, lasting weight loss is that people will not accept their true feelings about themselves and their weight. Instead, they fight their feelings, judge their feelings, try not to feel them, and basically criticize themselves for having those feelings in the first place. This is called repression, and what happens when you repress feelings is that you give them power out of all proportion, and they grow stronger and stronger until they take revenge. That's how human nature works. If you repress your feelings, if you reject or deny your feelings, they get stronger and stronger, and they'll cause you more and more trouble in your life. So if you want to make changes in your life, you really have no choice with your feelings. You have to acknowledge them, you have to accept them.

The self-hypnosis technique I'm going to show you now can teach you how to manage your feelings instead of having your feelings manage you. Some simple writing is involved, and I want you to do it with your non-dominant hand. Why? Because I want you to break out of your ordinary conscious mindset and respond more freely, creatively, as if you're a child again just learning to write.

Also, remember, if your self-hypnosis work ever feels like it's too much, or you feel overwhelmed in any way, do your breath work and go to the Second Watcher—you'll immediately feel more relaxed, aware, detached, and accepting.

So, with a pencil and pad of paper by your chair, do your normal trance preparation: Take several deep, satisfying breaths, accept your breathing as it is, then focus on the turning points. Be open to any personal imagery that might be brought up. As you feel yourself beginning to relax, your eyes growing heavy, or your hands tingling, settling into trance . . .

Now, I want you to focus on the whole issue of losing weight and keeping it off. It's been a big issue in your life for a long time. You've probably had some success and some failure, and you've probably dieted, probably started different programs. Well now we're going to start with accepting everything about your journey and all the feelings you have about it.

And the first thing, of course, is I want you to be aware of everything you feel. That's right. Okay, now with your nondominant hand, write down on the pad what you feel about this issue. It's fine if it looks like scribbling, doodling, or childlike writing. It's not going to be read by anyone or analyzed. Write down all the different feelings you have about losing weight and keeping it off. For example, do you feel doubtful? Do you feel frustrated? Do you feel judgmental? Do you feel hopeless? Guilty? Afraid? Sad? Make a list of all your feelings, and after you make the list, you're going to learn how to accept each one of these feelings because they are parts of you.

Now, let's begin a committee meeting about your feelings. Let's say you have seven different feelings about losing weight. Going back and forth between your dominant and non-dominant hands, draw seven circles and arrange them like chairs around a large round conference table. Write one of your feelings in each of the seven circles; these are your committee members, and they represent your seven different feelings about your weight loss problem. Finally, in the upper corner of the paper draw a large heart and write in it the word "Observer." This is your inner eye who acts as the committee chairperson, and who sees and accepts all your feelings without judgment or criticism. Have your Observer look at each circle, at each committee member, at each feeling, one at a time. Have your Observer consider each feeling, one after the other, with curiosity, compassion, and caring.

As your Observer looks carefully at each committee

member, you're learning how to accept your feelings, and thus how to accept yourself as you are. And you may notice that, with this attention, with this acceptance, your feelings will start to get smaller and smaller, shrink to their natural size, and become a lot more manageable.

Save the list of feelings you've scribbled in this session, because in the next chapter, on expression, I'm going to extend this trance and help you let each feeling express itself in its own voice. That's the next step in the healing process. But for now simply be aware of your feelings and accept them as they are.

You might be surprised. Just through awareness and acceptance, you'll find yourself changing and evolving. Later on today or tomorrow when you feel angry about being overweight (and you will), you might accept that a part of you feels angry. Then the next day when you start to feel hopeless about ever losing weight (and you will), you might accept that a part of you feels hopeless. And this will spread to other parts of your life. When something difficult or stressful happens, you'll accept it. Then when the stress disappears you'll accept that, too. When you feel good, you'll accept it. Then when the good feeling goes away, you'll accept that as well. You'll not be trying to change anything, fix anything, or get rid of anything. You'll be learning to observe and accept all your feelings just as they are.

The truth is that you're not going to get rid of your feelings anyway. You could spend one hundred years in counseling, you could take all the medication in the world, you could do every diet, every exercise program, you could do anything and everything and you're not going to get rid of your feelings.

You see, your feelings—all your feelings—are essential, organic parts of you, like your fingers and your toes. They've grown and developed with you through all the ages and stages of your life, as you've learned to get along with different people and to cope with different problems. When your fingers or toes are hurt or you bruise them, you don't cut them off and try and get rid of them; you take better care of yourself and you heal them. You're learning to do the same thing with your feelings.

Food Instead of Love

The whole issue of eating and overeating is intricately bound up with one of the most powerful of human feelings, love. We all have an innate need for love; studies have shown that infants will actually waste away and perish if they receive insufficient love and affectionate physical contact. At the same time, a deep association exists between love and food because we receive love and food together from our mother, or in some cultures, from our nurse. In fact, for most of us food becomes a positive trigger for feelings of love, nurturing, comfort, and safety, starting from the time we snuggle warm at the breast or the bottle and drink our fill. So, we all need love and we all intimately associate love with food.

Problems occur when, as we grow up, our steady source of love (mother *or* father) becomes uncertain or withheld for some reason (divorce, depression, alcohol or drug abuse are often the culprits). In this case, and because of the early association, we may fall back on food to give us the feeling of love that we're missing. In other words, food becomes a substitute for the love we need, and the deeper our need—or our hunger—for love, the more we eat.

In grievous cases, when a mother's or father's love is inappropriate, possibly abusive, the need for love can become bent and twisted into a vicious circle. We eat to feel loved and comforted, but we also eat to become so overweight that no one else will want to touch us. Then no one loves us (we've made sure of that), and so we eat even more to fill the emptiness—and round and round we go.

The only way out of these problems is to relax into awareness and accept your very natural human need for love. No matter how deep your need, accept your need for that much love. No matter how deeply troubled your experience of love, accept your need for better, more wholesome love. Don't hide or repress your need for love, don't try to need love less. By accepting your need for love, you'll get into a much healthier, more compassionate relationship with yourself, and you'll be able to love yourself well enough to make up for any deficiencies.

To help you understand how the relationship between love and food can become toxic in our lives, consider the case of Barbara.

When Barbara was six years old, she overheard an argument between her parents. She listened outside the bedroom door as her furious father threatened to leave the house for good. Little Barbara was terrified. She felt she must have done something very bad to make her father want to leave.

Later, when her mother found her in tears, Barbara was unable to explain why she was so upset. In her six-year-old mind, she thought her father would be mad if he knew she'd been eavesdropping, and then he'd surely leave. Even when her mother tried to cheer her up by taking her out for ice cream, Barbara was only partially comforted. Maybe, she worried, she'd done something so bad that her mother would leave her as well.

For weeks afterward Barbara tried to be on her best behavior, all the while living in fear of waking up an finding her parents gone. She became frantic if left alone for even a few minutes, and she was unable to express her fears. The only time she felt better was when her mother gave her something to eat.

Not surprisingly, this childhood fear of being abandoned because she was "bad," coupled with the reinforced association of food with her mother's love, led Barbara to become a chronic overeater and badly overweight as a young woman. She tried many, many diets, but the belief system she'd built up wouldn't allow her to make any positive change in her eating habits. She felt down deep that she was "bad," unlovable, and she had learned that eating meant love and security. And then the twist: Eating also made her so heavy that it was harder for anyone else to love her—or at least she believed that if someone loved her, fat as she was, he would "really" love her and not leave her.

When Barbara was thirty-three, she began instruction in self-hypnosis to overcome her food addiction. Her therapist helped her explore this critical childhood memory, and as she began to understand and accept how much more she needed love than food, she was able to start loving herself and changing her life.

Yin and Yang

There's another important reason why you should accept your feelings, even if you don't like them, or are ashamed of them. Feelings are always connected intimately with their opposite, like the yin and yang in Chinese philosophy. This means that when you reject negative feelings about your weight, you not only give those feelings power, you also weaken positive feelings that you approve of. Thus if you try hard not to feel hopeless about losing weight, you also weaken your sense of *hopefulness*. If you try to keep from feeling angry at your body, you also diminish your *compassion*. If you repress your fear of making a change in your eating habits, you actually undermine your *courage* to try.

The following is an extended meditation on accepting the two sides of yourself. Recite this to yourself in a relaxed state, as if in a half-trance.

Picture a river flowing in its banks.
The two banks are not separate or opposite things.
They are joined together underneath, at the river bottom.
And the two banks, joined in the depths, allow the river
    to flow.
But the conscious mind cannot think so deeply.

It thinks on surfaces, and so it thinks in extremes: this
    or that,
One bank or the other, good or bad, fat or skinny, overeat
    or don't eat.
It says, "If I'm going to be happy, I have to stop eating."
But you're working against yourself if you choose sides.
Be aware and accept that the two banks are part of the river,
And that the river flows swiftly because both banks hold
    strong.

People working hard on weight loss have told me, shaking
    their heads:
"Yesterday I was in control, and today I have almost none."
Well, control never happens by itself; loss of control is
    bound to follow.
Watch the waves at the beach; they do the same thing.
A really big set of waves is followed by a long lull.
So one day you're the big waves, the next day you're
    the lull.
So one day your will power is strong, the next day it's weak.
Where there are peaks, there are valleys.
Be aware and accepting of both.
Don't get stuck trying to be one or the other.
Enjoy the control while it lasts, and enjoy the loss of control
    when it comes.
Control is exciting but nobody can stay excited every
    moment of every day.
And what's wrong with losing control? It can be relaxing.
    And fun.

Breathing is not all inhales or exhales, it's not either . . . or.
It's the union of the two that creates the flow of breath.
The breath comes in and the breath goes out—
You have a rhythm, and it's the rhythm that keeps you alive.
Your unconscious mind paces this rhythm.

It's the master of inner rhythm and balance and union.
It knows when to breathe in, and when to breathe out.
And it maintains the rhythm even when your conscious
    mind is asleep.
Trust your unconscious and enjoy both your inhale and
    your exhale.
It's no good choosing one or the other.
Life is in the balance.

Not Perfect, but Perfectly Okay

We all make mistakes, but few of us really accept them and
learn from them. How many times have you tried dieting? Each
time it didn't last. And you probably blamed yourself. Was I too
weak? Was I too lazy? The real mistake—and it guaranteed you
wouldn't reach your goals—was in not accepting yourself, in
not loving yourself as you are. And as with all love denied, food
becomes the consolation.

Here's a meditation to help you think about how you blame
and limit yourself—beat yourself up—with self-criticism. Take
several deep breaths and feel your body relaxing. When you're
getting a little dreamy, read this softly and slowly to yourself . . .

You carry around the expectation of perfection.
When you make mistakes, which of course happens daily,
You reject yourself, you judge yourself,
And make yourself miserable with self-criticism.
Self-condemned, you grab for something to save you,
    soothe you—often food.
But when you accept yourself, love yourself,
Your perspective is much bigger, and the need to eat is not
    there.
So accept that you're not perfect—but that you're
    perfectly okay.

Learn to love yourself and accept yourself as you are,
  mistakes and all.
Don't wait for the future, hoping you'll achieve perfection
  some day.
Don't let the life you have slip by because it's imperfect.
Start accepting your mistakes now, and start enjoying your
  life now.
With acceptance that you're not perfect, but perfectly okay,
Your body can start losing weight.
The more you enjoy life, the less you'll overeat.
A really happy person feels full inside.

Look on the Lighter Side

We all take ourselves, our mistakes, and our problems way
too seriously sometimes. If we could only step back and realize
how funny, silly—even how ridiculous—we're being as we try to
cope with life, we might be able to lighten up on our self-criticism
and stop playing the blame game.

Try this Second Watcher trance to get in touch with the hu-
morous side of your eating. Breathe, relax, and drift into self-
hypnosis. When you're ready . . .

> *Now from the last row of the theater, how do you want
> scenes about losing weight and keeping it off to go in your
> movie? This is the best place to write the script. So from
> the last row of the theater, I want you to rehearse the movie
> the way you want it to go, losing weight, eating, dealing
> with stressful social situations, sexual relationships, issues
> at work, conversations eye-to-eye with family members.
> Anything you want to work through. From the last row of
> the theater, you're writing the script of how the movie is
> going to go, and you're doing it by rehearsing the scenes, by
> trying different approaches.*

But this time you may decide to make the movie a comedy. Maybe if you have a sense of humor today, you'll actually write the script so that everything goes wrong in the craziest ways. Not that it's going to go that way in the final version of the movie, but just so you can laugh, and trip over your own feet, stumble and fall, and kind of get that stress out of the way.

Have you seen those "blooper" shows on TV, or the out-takes added onto some comedy DVDs? You know, the clips showing the actors forgetting their lines, stumbling on words, and cracking each other up? Or the painting falling off the wall during the scene, or the prop chair not breaking in the fight when it's supposed to? And the actors come out of their roles, come out of the scene, look at the camera, and dissolve in laughter. Make your own blooper show of the comic "mis-takes" for your movie. Let yourself laugh at the comic side of your eating and dieting.

I hope you can see that "working" on your weight problems can be fun, playful, creative, intuitive, and relaxing. (And you thought it was all about calories, fat, carbs, work-outs, and suffering.)

Hug Your Child

Like your feelings and the mistakes you've made, your past is something you can't get rid of. It's with you always, an in-grained part of you. It's like the rings of a tree—you know, the growth rings inside a tree that reflect each year's climatic conditions. In any tree's life, some years were more difficult than others, and so some of its rings are narrow for the drought years, while some are wide for the years of ample rain.

Now if a tree isn't doing well, you can't cut it down and carve out the rings for the difficult years, and then glue it back together and expect it to grow. Good or bad, narrow or wide, those rings have been an integral part of the tree's growth and development. They are the tree.

Well, you are like a tree. You cannot change the experiences in your past. But what you *can* do is accept your past and learn from it how to take better care of yourself now and in the future.

In the following trance your present gets in touch with your past for a powerful moment of self-acceptance. As always, get your breath going, and remember that if you ever want to feel safe and comfortable, you know how to become the Second Watcher . . .

Good. Now you're going to take a long, relaxing walk. That's right, and remember the past is always behind you and the future is always in front of you.

As you begin your walk, notice that you're on a great, beautiful pathway, wide enough for plenty of people to pass, but that you're the only one walking today. And as you continue walking and going down a little hill, you can see the graceful trees growing and all the branches where they spread out over the pathway almost creating a canopy. A truly beautiful place. You can see the birds, but you can hear them more than see them. You can see the blue sky through the branches of the trees, feel the sun's warmth. Just an absolutely perfect day. And here you are, with this area to yourself, and it's really safe, really beautiful. Mother Nature has been very generous to this spot.

And as you continue walking down the hill, you notice that way, way down the hill there's a very big tree. It looks like it might be the biggest tree in the whole forest. And you're interested in it and walk toward it, and you notice some squirrels in the distance running up the tree branches. The clouds are looking really pretty up there, way up in the sky. It's one of those days that you just love because it's so comfortable, nature is so bounteous. And you're continuing to walk toward the tree, and as you get closer and closer, you realize there's a small person sitting right at the base of the tree, down by the roots of the tree. Curious. And so you walk closer and closer, and as you do, you realize that the young person looks kind of familiar. And as you get closer and closer, and get right up to this young child, you realize this young child is you. What a powerful moment. And the child and you reach out to each other and hold each other, and hug each other, and you feel the closeness and the oneness, maybe in a way neither of you has felt for a long, long time. You both have this great feeling of love, and care, and deep connection. Wow, it's a magical moment.

And now a conversation can happen where the present you says everything you want to say to the child, any advice, any encouragement, any warnings, any mention of gifts or talents. And of course, the young child listens, totally open to whatever you want to express. Yes, that's right.

And naturally, the young child wants to say some things to you, some advice, some warnings, a mention of some gifts, some encouragement. And of course, you listen, fully open to the child's words. That's right. What a beautiful interaction. What a great experience that you can come back to anytime.

Soon you realize the sun is getting low, and it's time to walk back up the hill, back to where you started. And as you do, you feel different, more connected to yourself if that's possible. More alive, and refreshed, and relaxed if that's possible, with a great sense of relief and encouragement. And you notice even more colors walking back, and more trees, and shapes in the clouds, and just a world of difference in how much more clearly you see things.

This is a trance to visit many times, so that you can encounter yourself at the pivotal ages or stages of your weight problems—maybe the five-year-old you, or the ten-year-old, or the fifteen-year-old; maybe when you began to gain weight, or when you were first teased about being fat, or when you first related your weight with your sexuality. Or any time you just need a hug.

Deprogramming Your Eating Habits

To a large extent, we've all been shaped by our past, programmed by our experiences, imprisoned by our habits. Once you've done any habit—like overeating—for a long time, it takes root in your body. It's in your chemistry. It becomes automatic.

In order to free yourself from your eating habits, you need to de-automatize, deprogram yourself. A deprogrammed eater is naturally thin. But the process does not involve slaving, starving, and dieting—eating unappetizing food that someone says is good for you. The secret to changing your eating habits is to live in the moment with awareness and acceptance.

This meditation can help you understand what I mean. Take three deep, refreshing breaths and read this aloud:

When you walk, walk slowly . . . watch.
When you look, look with clarity . . . observe.
The trees, you'll see,
Are greener than they've ever been.
When you listen, listen closely . . . attend.
The birds, you'll hear,
Sing more sweetly than you can imagine.
Learn something, too.
Learn awareness and acceptance.
Let the moment be your purpose,
Focus on the moment at hand.

Accept the voices that try to block the way—
"You'll never be thin," and "It's too hard."
Don't repress or they'll fight back stronger.
Just observe and be polite.
Never say, "I hate you, go away!"
Say, "Yes, I hear you. Thank you.
But I choose not to follow you."

Body Perspectives

A vital issue in losing weight is body image—what you see when you look at your body, and what you feel about what you see. If you love your body, you live in it, you take care of it, and you don't stuff it with unnecessary food. But if you reject your body, you become indifferent and negligent, because who cares about the enemy? You'll not look at it, you'll apologize for it, you'll stop listening to its messages—and you'll hate it even more.

How do you develop a positive body image? How do you learn to accept your body, and so break the cycle of self-judgment/self-hatred that drives your overeating? Here's a body-acceptance exercise that has much the same effect as a Second Watcher trance:

Stand nude or in your underwear in front of a full-length mirror and look at your whole body; from face to feet. Be aware of your feelings as you do this. Perhaps you'll like some parts of what you see more than others. Most people find some parts difficult and unacceptable, because they frustrate or dissatisfy them. But overweight people are severely self-critical. Perhaps you see a chubbiness in your face you don't want to deal with. Perhaps you hate your stomach or your thighs so much that you can barely stand to look at them. Perhaps you see signs of obesity and you can't bear to stay connected with the thoughts and feelings these signs evoke. So the reaction is to escape—to repress your feelings, to judge, reject, deny, disown, and try not to be parts of yourself.

Rather than look away, however, try to stay focused on your body image for just a few more minutes. Keep looking in the mirror, do your breath work, and try saying to yourself, "I accept my body as it is. I am 100% friendly, caring and compassionate towards my body."

Now let's experiment with perspective.

First, step up to the mirror so close that you're almost touching the glass. Notice that your head and especially your nose and eyes are large all out of proportion. You can hardly even see your body. You likely feel grotesque and ugly—it's a hall of mirrors experience—and you can easily reject this image.

Next, take a step or two back. You can see your whole body now, but you're so close to the image that it's easy to pick out your body's flaws and exaggerate them—and then to judge and criticize yourself.

Finally, step way back—say about ten feet back—and now you can see the full picture of yourself. You're a whole human being with your own unique body, and also with your own personal spirit, energy, warmth, and style.

Just remember: Each of these three images in the mirror is you. It's simply a matter of having a different perspective, seeing things with different eyes, and seeing the bigger picture.

Do this exercise for one minute every morning and one minute every night. The benefits are extraordinary. Within a few days you'll begin to find a new and more positive body image. Plus, you'll become more accepting of your whole self, which will then help you grow in self-confidence and self-respect.

Also, once you've learned to accept your body as it is now, you'll be more motivated to take better care of yourself and improve your eating and exercise habits. As in all relationships, the better you feel about the person, the more you want to do for them. Of course, the opposite is true, too; the more judging or frustrated or angry you are with another person, the less you want to do for them. And so the relationship with your own body, when it's accepting and loving, can be the driving force behind your desire to lose weight and keep it off.

And lastly, your willingness to see and accept yourself as you are will work wonders in all your relationships. When you're more comfortable with yourself, you're more comfortable with others. When you can laugh at yourself, you can laugh more easily with your friends. And only when you love yourself with no strings attached do you have the freedom to truly love another person.

Tree Roots

Accepting your body can mean more than just being comfortable with how it looks. There's an even bigger picture, an even larger context of acceptance. You might also come to understand that this is the body nature has given you. It was not created to make you suffer and have you reject it. No animal thinks it's fat and hates itself because of its body—not even the hippopotamus. No plant suffers and rejects itself for being too big—not even a giant redwood. This is the body you have, this is the body nature has given you. Use it, enjoy it, and care for it as nature intended.

To help you experience your body's deep connection to nature, I want to take you on another relaxing walk. First take some deep, cleansing breaths and drift into a dreamy trance . . .

When you take a walk outside, and maybe this is one of the things you do to relieve stress, you notice how beautiful the trees are, and certainly it feels as if you're seeing the trees with different eyes and with some clarity. Maybe you've already done your breathing, maybe you're doing your breathing as you walk. Either way, walking and breathing, breathing and walking, you notice that the trees you see in your mind's eye are as much a part of existence as you are, and you're as much as the trees are.

To demonstrate this to you, and to have some fun with this self-hypnosis session, put your feet flat on the floor or the ground. Go ahead and change positions if you have to, just make sure you get both feet flat on the floor or the ground. And as you do this be aware of the feelings in your feet, that's right, give all your attention to the feelings in your feet. Your heels, the balls of your feet, your toes. That's right. Whether you have shoes on, or socks, or bare feet, just be aware of your feet. Try to be your feet.

And as you put all your attention, all your focus, into your feet, you may notice some interesting sensations, maybe some heaviness, maybe some tingling. That's right. Just allow what's happening to happen. There's nothing you have to try to do, there's nothing you have to fight. You're learning how to take the best possible care of yourself, from your feet up. That's right, energy always moves up. Good.

Now with your feet flat on the floor or ground, it's time to imagine that your feet actually have roots going into the earth. Feel the roots coming out of the bottom of your feet into the earth, they go down into the earth maybe a foot, two feet, three feet, four feet, five feet. Depending on how old or young you feel as a tree, allow the roots to come right out of your feet, go right into the earth and feel them branching out into the earth. That's right. So you have a feeling of being grounded, being connected, being part of the earth, and certainly rooted deeply into the experience of life. And so anytime you want to feel grounded, want to feel strongly connected to life, just put all your awareness into your feet

*just as you're doing now. That's right. Feel it, visualize it,
let yourself experience it.*

*What you'll find is that whenever you're walking or
standing outside, you'll be able to feel grounded, feel the
roots coming right out of your feet, and you'll enter a
beautiful state of relaxation just by putting your awareness
into your feet and feeling grounded. You can do this sitting
down, you can do this walking. You can carry this with you
everywhere you go. This is one of the beautiful gifts you
can have with you all the time.*

The healing power of feeling rooted, part of the earth,
grounded in nature, is that you're continually reconnecting yourself to what really matters. You're alive. You're part of life. You're
bigger than your problems. You're deeper and more rooted than
the issues around weight, food, and exercise.

Losing weight and keeping it off happens naturally when
you get out of your conscious mind and feel more alive and well
in your body. Enjoy yourself. Enjoy your awareness and acceptance. Enjoy your body, feet first.

Thank Your Body

Your body is a wonder of nature. It's an incredible organism,
so complex and yet so efficient that it goes on functioning for
seventy years or more. Whether you're awake or asleep, aware
or unaware, it goes on working, goes on being of service to you.
Even without you knowing or caring, it goes about its business
of breathing, pumping blood, processing food, building and replacing cells, on and on. Without help from your conscious
mind, and often in spite of your ego's interference, your body
goes on giving you the gift of life.

It's time to be grateful. It's time for a thank-you card.

Get yourself as comfortable as possible, maybe stretch out a little bit and focus on your breath work. Maybe you have an awareness of the turning points where your inhale turns into an exhale, and your exhale turns into an inhale. Perhaps you're having some fun with colors, breathing them in and breathing them out. Maybe you're going to a favorite place, a place you love that's always welcoming, that's always peaceful. Maybe you're on the mountain watching yourself relax, or maybe you're in the last row of the theater watching the movie of your life, and from the Second Watcher perspective feeling more and more friendliness, compassion, and caring for yourself. When you're ready . . .

> *Take this moment to communicate to yourself, right now, just three little lines and say these to your body out loud:*
>
> *"Thank you for working so well for me all these years. I'm sorry if I've been ignoring you. If there's anything that you're trying to tell me, I'm totally open right now."*
>
> *Now I want you to repeat these lines, say these lines aloud one more time, while you focus on that part of your body where there's tension or any kind of stress: "Thank you for working so well for me all these years. I'm sorry if I've been ignoring you. If there's anything you're trying to tell me, I'm totally open right now."*
>
> *Beautiful. You can do this as often as you wish. Like all these skills, you could never practice this too much.*

Gaining Insight

You can also become more accepting of your body—and yourself—by learning to see and to accept objects on their own terms. Everything around you has its own unique existence, its own properties, qualities, its own integrity. The lamp by your chair has its own size and color, its own structure and function, its own history, as well as its own essential "lampness," a character all its own. If you practice seeing objects as they are, as existing in their own right—this might be called "object-ivity" training—you'll begin to accept how unique and beautiful you are yourself.

Go ahead and begin with your breathing if you haven't already. Be aware of the rise and fall of each breath, accept your breathing as it is, and be aware of the turning points. Naturally, I want you to get as comfortable as possible. Don't concentrate, just relax, simple awareness, nothing is rejected . . .

Now give all of your attention totally to one object. Find an object wherever you are and focus your attention on this one object. It might be something you look at all the time, or something you hardly ever notice. Just concentrate on it, just keep watching it. Don't blink your eyes because blinking gives space to losing attention. And as you keep watching, concentrating on this one object, it may even look like it's dissolving right in front of your eyes. You don't want to miss a moment, so it's important not to blink your eyes. That's right.

And as you're looking at this one object, look at it lovingly now with all your attention totally on this one object. Look at it with loving feelings, with some admiration, with some positive intentions, with kindness, with friendliness, with caring, with compassion. Look at the object as a whole object, a whole thing. Now look at the object as if you're seeing it for the very first time. That's right. Perhaps to your own surprise you find that you can see into the center of the object like this. Into its very core.

It's fun to see how, with your eyes open, just by changing your focus and refocusing a little, you can see things so differently. It's like a secret. Giving all your attention totally to one object, concentrating on it, and maybe even dissolving it, and not blinking your eyes because blinking loses attention. You look lovingly at this object, friendly, caring, compassionate. You look at the object as a whole, and as if it were the very first time. And you can enter into the center of the object.

Okay, here's the secret. Once you can do this with an object, you can do this with other people—and you can even do this with yourself. That's right. You can enter your own center by doing this. And once you know your center, you can feel at home within yourself. So once you can do it with an object, giving all of your attention to this one object, you can do this with yourself. You can enter your center like this. Look lovingly, look at yourself as a whole, even look at yourself as if for the very first time. Once you know the center, you can feel at home within yourself.

The more you can see into yourself lovingly, with 100 percent awareness and acceptance, the simpler it will be for you to eat intelligently, to be more physically active, and to enjoy the journey as well as the results.

Accept Others as They Are

If you can learn to accept objects as they are, you can do the same thing with other people. This is perhaps even more important, because when you judge and reject others, you automatically distance and estrange yourself from them. And as I've explained, when your personal relationships are not close and loving, not "ful-filling," you will often fill yourself with food as a substitute.

Now it's pretty clear that judging others is a pretty useless business in the first place. The old saying, "You can't judge a book by its cover," is even more true about people. You simply can't tell what's inside a person by seeing his or her face. The real person is usually in hiding, and so chances are your judgment is going to be wrong. For instance, you've heard of the happy fat person. Well, in most cases overweight persons smile on the surface, while deep inside they are sad and hurting—they are in fact smiling to hide wounds or scars that would be embarrassing if made public.

It's easier to judge people by what they do, but here again people's public acts are usually motivated by private issues that you know nothing about. You know this is true because when people judge you by your actions—say, your eating habits—you feel that they've judged you wrongly. It's as if they've clipped a single scene out of your movie and judged the whole movie by it. It's not right, it's out of context. Your real story is totally different.

So rather than judging and criticizing people and their actions, you need to go deeper and learn to be more accepting of them. Of course, you mustn't *try* to stop judging people; trying to stop would just mean that you're judging yourself for judging others, and that would get you nowhere. Instead, become aware and accept the fact that you're in the habit of judging people.

The Second Watcher technique can help. Breathe and relax into a trance as you would normally, see yourself sitting in the fifteenth row watching the movie of your life . . .

Now imagine that you're in the last row of the theater, watching the watcher in the fifteenth row, and both of you are watching the movie. Only this time you see on the screen a person you know quite well, and whom you tend to criticize a lot, maybe a colleague at work, maybe your boss, maybe a neighbor, maybe your spouse at home. That's right, someone in your life whom you're quick to judge.

While you're watching this person acting in your movie, acting as they always do, imagine that the screen gets wavy

*for a second and there's a flashback to this person's child-
hood, maybe to when they were five or six years old. Good.
See if you can tell what the person looked like as a youngster; listen to what they sounded like, imagine what their
home life was like, their parents, their brothers or sisters.
Give yourself some time to make the scene as detailed as
possible.*

*The screen gets wavy again and the movie flashes for-
ward to a time when the person you judge so severely is old,
maybe eighty or eighty-five years old. Here again, see if
you can imagine what this person will look like in their later
years, what they'll sound like, who'll be left in their life,
what they'll do with their time. That's right.*

*The screen gets wavy once again and you return to the
present day. Look at this person you judge, at how they
look now, acting in your movie, and see if you can get a
glimpse of the five-year-old in the present person. Maybe
the nose is the same, maybe a look in the eye, maybe how
they walk. See the child hiding in the grown-up. Now look
again and see if you can find the eighty-year-old in the
present person. It's the same person, only maybe the shoulders have stooped, the voice has thinned, or the walk has
slowed. See the elder in the grown-up.*

*And now from the Second Watcher, or whenever you're
ready, ask yourself, after having this experience, how do you
feel about the movie? After having this experience, how do
you feel about the person you judge?*

Speak Your Name

On one of my journeys of teaching and learning, I was in India and I was introduced to a lady who had been a house cleaner
for about fifty-five years. One day she had an epiphany and
realized that she had healing hands and was meant to be teach-

ing yoga. Well everybody thought that this was crazy, but she listened to herself and within about two years she had become one of the most sought-after healers in all of India. Which is really saying something, because there are a lot of wonderful healers in India.

So I went to meet this lady and of course I asked the questions I often ask when I meet very healing and wonderful people. What's the meaning of life? You know, simple questions like that. And, what's your most useful technique for relaxation, meditation, self-hypnosis? She told me that the most important thing in life was patience. And then she taught me this self-healing technique. It was her gift to me, and now I'm giving it to you.

If your eyes haven't already grown heavy, please let them. Make yourself as comfortable as possible . . .

> *Go through your breathing, any imagery of a favorite place, maybe the Second Watcher perspective, maybe breathing colors, maybe doing some progressive relaxation to release any tension in your body. Perhaps remembering the past is always behind you, the future is always in front of you. You're always in the present. Focus on your breathing again, inhale and exhale, just simply focusing, inhale and then exhale.*
>
> *On the exhale say your own name to yourself, but not out loud, just say your own name. So you inhale and on the exhale you say your own name to yourself, and continue doing this for the next minute or so. You're not used to hearing yourself say your own name, certainly not repeatedly. You have a certain response to your name usually when other people say it. Watch what happens. Stay with it repeating your own name to yourself. If you get distracted, because most people do, just keep coming back to your name and saying it on the exhale.*

You're going to want to practice this for a minute or two, or five minutes, whenever you have a chance. Maybe when you sit down to read the paper, just take a few minutes first, close your eyes, focus on your breath work and any other techniques that relax you. Then inhale and on the exhale say your own name.

You might be asking (along with Shakespeare's Juliet), "What's in a name?" Perhaps quite a bit. Ancient people believed that a person's name was more than a label; the name not only told the origin and lineage of the person, but it also held the spirit, the essence, the true identity of the person.

Maybe without knowing it, the Indian healer I met had tapped into the self-healing power of embracing your own name. Give her technique some time and energy, and watch what happens. You'll be pleasantly surprised.

You Can't Please Everyone

By studying the meditations and practicing the trance ideas you find in this chapter, your relationship with your body and with your self will become stronger and more accepting. And as this happens, you'll realize how important it is just to be yourself and not get too caught up worrying about what other people think of you.

Besides, you know, it really doesn't matter. No matter what you look like, whether you're tall or short, big or small, fat or thin, dark or light, strong or weak, about a third of people are going to think you're great, about a third of people are hardly going to notice you, and about a third of people aren't going to like you. It's always been this way and always will be. It's called the "One/Third Theory."

And what if you try really hard to make everybody like you? Sorry, it's still going to be the "One/Third Theory." About a third of people will appreciate your efforts and like you. Another third will be too busy to notice. And a third won't like you because you're trying so hard to please everyone.

So, don't try to make your life what you think it *should* be to get more people to like you or approve of you. Consider the "One/Third Theory" and be yourself, accept yourself, love yourself—just as you are.

CHAPTER 11

Phase Three: Expression

Awareness unlocks the door. Acceptance opens the door and starts you on your way. But you still have an important part of the journey to take before you can be truly free of your chronic overeating and yo-yo dieting. Your goal, your destination, is to be healthier and happier in your life, and therefore in your relationship with food. The next step on the pathway, and the next phase in the Keep It Off Weight-loss Program, is Expression.

By "Expression" I mean taking the material you've been uncovering and accepting in the last two chapters, all the memories, family issues, thoughts, habits—and the many feelings you've had about all these things—and releasing them, letting them go, literally pushing them out, or "ex-pressing" them. Remember, it was repression—denying these feelings, hiding from them, holding them in, pushing them down into your body—that put your emotional weight on in the first place. And you've been struggling ever since with the physical weight that came along with it. Well, expressing is the opposite of repressing, and now it's time to open up, give voice to your feelings, and let them go.

The expression you're going to give to your feelings in this chapter will sometimes be spoken, sometimes written, sometimes non-verbal, but in any case it will be a private matter, not communicated openly to other persons (such as a parents), no matter how implicated they might be in your eating and weight problems. I've found that 90 percent of the time you can deal with your issues and express your feelings in your trance work, or in confidential exercises, and resolve them just fine, without ever having to confront other people personally.

A couple of cautions: Expressing your feelings doesn't mean blurting them out right in the moment whenever you feel something. As long as you're aware of your feelings and accept them, you can wait and express them later, when you're doing your self-hypnosis or performing a letting-go exercise. Nor should you overdo your expressiveness. You don't need to let go all day with every feeling. Express your feelings at most two or three times a day, and only on the big issues. By learning the techniques and doing the exercises in this chapter, you'll be able to express yourself and release your feelings in a healthy, organized, and empowering way and then let it rest a while.

I post these small caution signs because the self-expression you're going to be practicing in this chapter feels so good that it's easy to get carried away with it. When you're letting go of your repressed feelings, it's as if they're uncoiling, or surging up, bubbling up, with a lot of new energy. You might feel weightless, as if a burden has disappeared, or you might feel at ease, calmed down, slowed down. But you'll always feel very, very alive, rejuvenated, as if years have disappeared and you're younger, livelier, fresher.

Letting It Go

Here are two techniques to help get you warmed up mentally and physically for the process of letting go. The first is a guided visualization, and the second is a much more active expressiveness exercise.

Imagine all your worries, frustrations, negative thoughts and feelings—your emotional and mental weight—packed tightly into a small, stuffy, sour smelling room. Picture yourself opening a window in that room. A fresh breeze blows in, so clear and cool it opens all your senses, and all the negatives swirl and drift out into the fresh air. Take three deep, satisfying breaths and relax.

It almost seems as if fat adheres to repressed emotions. So to lose weight and keep it off you sometimes have to fight to get your feelings out.

Have a special pillow, or maybe even buy a punching bag. For ten minutes each morning get hold of your pillow, or put on your boxing gloves, and let all your feelings go. Hit the pillow or the body bag, bite it, kick it, hug it, throw it. Let everything come out. All the anger, sadness, resentment, or guilt—whatever you've felt all these years about being overweight. Say what you need to say, shout, sob, scream. Hold nothing back.

Then for ten more minutes, sit silently and relax deeply. Love your *self*. It's time to learn to set yourself free. Like a bird let out of a cage. Fly!

The Committee Meeting, Part 3

The Committee Meeting technique is an organized and comprehensive way to express all of your many (and often conflicting) thoughts and feelings about losing weight and keeping it off.

As in the committee meeting for acceptance in Chapter 10, I want you to write certain things down in this session, and I want you to use your non-dominant hand. This will help free you from your social programming and allow your intuitive, unconscious mind to express itself. Also, bring along the list you made in Chapter 10 of the various feelings, or the different parts of you—the various committee members—you need to hear from concerning your weight. Doubtful, Frustrated, Guilty, Sad, your Inner Child, your Inner Parent, your Physical Self, your Spiritual Self, on and on. You know who they are.

Let me remind you that if the feelings in this trance get to be too much, too stressful, or you just need a break at anytime during your committee meeting, you can always use your breathing and get yourself up to the Second Watcher perspective, to the top of the mountain or the last row of the theater, from where you can look on more calmly and with more detachment.

So get yourself comfortably into trance. Breathe deeply and focus on the turning points. Feel your arms or legs tingling. See yourself walking down a flight of carpeted stairs to the committee room . . .

> *And in a minute but not yet, we're going over to the conference table. It's a big circular table, of highly polished wood, and there are different committee members sitting around the table. Each one of the committee members represents a different part of you, a different feeling, maybe a different age or stage in your life. And maybe you already know the name of the first committee member. If you need to peek at your list, you can.*
>
> *So whenever you're ready, take your seat in the corner of the room and let this healing and freeing process begin. You know the issue, you know what you're working on, and with your non-dominant hand and just allowing it to move across the paper, give the first committee member a voice. Give the first committee member, whether it's Angry or Afraid or Guilty, whatever it is, from your heart to your head to your hand, time to express its feelings. Maybe there's anger at yourself for being fat, or at others for being thin. Maybe there's fear of failing again, or of succeeding this time. Maybe you're guilty that you sneak food, or*

that you have hateful thoughts. No matter what it is, allow the feelings. Allow that this is how a part of you feels about being overweight.

Doodling, drawing, scribbling, words, pictures. You're allowing this part of you to express itself at last. Finally this committee member can express whatever it feels about your weight. No more pushing down. No more holding back. Accepting and letting go. Accepting and letting go. That's right. That's right.

No more repressing, no more holding back. Let yourself be completely and unconditionally accepting of this committee member, as though it's a child who really needs to be accepted. Who needs to be listened to. Who needs to get it all out.

It's okay. It's okay. From your heart to your head to your hand.

When you're ready, when you feel you've heard everything that this committee member feels, go to the next committee member and listen to what he or she has to say about eating. Go at your own pace. There's no rush. There's no race. If you need to peek at the name of the next committee member, that's fine. If you can tell who needs to speak next, that's fine too. Just let go, let go. Accepting everything this committee member feels and expresses about your weight, without judging, without filtering, without holding back. That's right.

Without any judgment, without any criticism, accepting and expressing. Accepting and letting go. That's right. And then go to the next committee member. Continue with your own evolution till you get all the way around your whole committee, one at a time. Maybe there's a ten-year-old you ("I really want a hamburger, fries, and a coke"), or a fifteen-year-old you ("I hate myself I look so fat"), or a twenty-year-old you ("Nobody's going to hire a fat person"). Maybe there's an adult you ("I've got to start getting in shape"), *or a parent you* (*"You need to take responsibility for your weight"*). *That's right. Accepting each one, one at a time. Expressing all the feelings. All the thoughts, all the pictures, all the words, all the silence, that's right. Finally you have this opportunity. It may even feel like you've been waiting for years and years. You have the opportunity right here, right now to give each committee member a voice, to be accepted, expressed, and released. That's right. And it feels right to be accepted and to express. It feels honorable and honest and truthful and freeing. That's right.*

And as you accept and express, you'll discover immediately and forever after how much lighter you feel emotionally, how much lighter you feel as a person, how much better you feel about how you're taking care of yourself from this day forward.

This is the bridge between your emotions and your mind, yes. And this frees you up in your heart and it frees you up in your head, both at the same time. That's right. Letting go, letting go, letting go. Accepting, expressing, letting go. There's no more holding back, no more pushing down. That's right.

Go all the way around so all the committee members have a chance to be accepted and to have their say. It's so freeing, just this alone is incredibly freeing and you'll see how this helps you tonight, tomorrow, the rest of the week, through the weekend, the rest of the month, the rest of the year and for years and years and years in the future, just this one experience now and learning how to take care of yourself . . . and letting go. Just keep letting go. Keep opening the doors to releasing and expressing. That's right.

The Committee Meeting technique is so important in all phases of self-hypnosis because it gives you an effective way to manage your throng of committee members. You can't fire them, you know. You can manage your committee members and they can get smaller, quieter, and feel more a part of the team; but there isn't any technique anywhere that will let you get rid of them. As you know, if you try to dominate your feelings they get stronger and stronger until they come to dominate you. So you're stuck with your committee members. But you don't have to be stuck in committee with them. If you become aware of your feelings, accept them, and express them—give them a strong voice and a proper hearing—you'll feel better and lighter within a few minutes.

It's the same with your thoughts. You'll always think and you'll always have negative, critical thoughts. You can't stop yourself from thinking negatively and, if you try, you only end up being more negative and self-critical. But when you become aware of your negative thoughts, accept them as they are, and express them to yourself, you feel relaxed and peaceful within a few minutes.

So, you can manage your feelings/thoughts/committee members, or they can manage you. Use the Committee Meeting trance as often as you like. It's simple. It's natural. It's self-hypnosis at its best.

Finish Your Unfinished Business

When I was a kid, people said that "Time heals all wounds." And today people say, pretty glibly, "Deal with it!" and "Get over it!" Well, I'm afraid that just doesn't happen very easily for most of us. I've worked with many, many elderly people, people in their eighties, and they're still struggling with negative, hurtful things that happened to them when they were children or teenagers. They've gotten on with their lives, one way or another, but they still have old wounds that haven't healed properly and are causing them trouble. In other words, they still have unfinished business to deal with, and as long as it's *un*finished, it continues to cause them inner conflict, stress, and health problems.

Of course, not everyone's issues date from childhood. You might have unfinished business concerning weight loss from just a few years, weeks, or days ago. But the point is that, to get healthy in your relationship with food and with yourself, you need to become aware of the hurts you've received, and understand how you've repressed your feelings about them.

And then begin to let them go.

Here's an extended variation of the Second Watcher trance that can help you give your feelings a voice and bring some release. Take several deep breaths, your eyes growing heavy, and remember the theater . . . you've been here before. Remember sitting in the fifteenth row, in the middle of the theater, then moving to the last row and watching yourself in the fifteenth row . . .

> *This is where we begin, sitting in a theater, only this time it's an auditorium, not a movie theater. Maybe you can see the stage. Maybe you can feel the hot stage lights. Maybe you can hear the actor's voices. I just want you to give yourself the experience of being in a theater, being in the last row, in the Second Watcher perspective. And you're watching way down there on the stage a scene in the play of your own life. I want you to remember what it feels like to be the Second Watcher, being in the last row, feeling detached, feeling comfortable, because if at any time during this work it feels like it's too much, you can always use your breathing as a bridge. Get yourself all the way back to the last row so you can feel safe, feel comfortable. It's always just a breath away.*
>
> *Now whenever you're ready, I want you to imagine that you walk down the aisle of the theater, all the way up to the stage, up the steps on the side. And when you get up on the stage you see that there's a person or maybe more than one person whom you know, and with whom you*

want to finish some unfinished business. Whoever that person is or whoever those people are, you organize the stage the way you want it. You can be sitting or standing. They can be on the other side of the stage or close by. You can have them sitting or standing. It's up to you. You design the set. You choreograph the movement. You make it any way you want it, the way you're most comfortable.

Now, I want you to imagine saying exactly what you feel to this person or to these people, whatever you feel about the way they've treated you, and as you're saying it, I want you to write it down with your non-dominant hand. Here's your opportunity. No more holding back. No more pushing down. Take this opportunity to let go, to express, to release whatever you feel towards this person or towards these people. That's right. Speaking, shouting, screaming, scribbling, doodling, writing words, expressing feelings. That's right.

This is all about you having the opportunity now to say whatever you want to say, whatever you've been holding back, whatever you've been wanting to express, whatever you've never said but knew you wanted to. Years of feelings, maybe decades of feelings, and you can now tell this other person or these other people how they've affected your life, what they've done to your life, what they've done to your self-esteem or to your relationships or to your weight.

So no more holding back. This is your time. This is your chance to accept whatever you feel, and the other person or people just have to sit there or stand there and listen, and you get to say everything, everything. And I'm going to give you time to express it all. I'm going to give you some encouragement to really let go. That's right.

If it's sad, let it be sad. If it's angry, let it be angry. If it's intense, let it be intense. If it's simple, let it be simple. If it's exactly what you thought you felt, wonderful. If it's different from what you thought you felt, now that you're *saying it, fine. It's all about you releasing, letting go. That's right.*

And what else do you want to express? Say it from your heart to your head to your hand. Let go. Release. Finally, finally. You've been waiting for this. You've been waiting to let go, probably for a very, very long time and now you have a safe and healing and empowering way to do it. Finally let go. That's right.

Let go, let go, let go. Finally it's your turn to finish with all the unfinished business. Everything you've been holding in your body, everything you've been holding in your head, everything that's been affecting you in so many ways. Accepting everything you feel and letting go. This is the path to freedom. This is the path to healing.

From your heart to your head to your hand, years of holding this in, months, days, minutes, moments, or it may feel like hundreds of years, like forever. You're saying what you need to say to the person or persons you need to say it to. You're being 100 percent responsible, 100 percent honest, 100 percent freeing of all these feelings you've been carrying around inside and you're letting them go right now.

That's right. That's right. Once and for all, let go. Out of your body, out of you directly to them and on to the paper, released out of your body. Free yourself up. Stop using your strength to hold it in. Get it out so you can use your strength for healthier and better things in your life from this day forward. That's right.

Take a few more minutes to let go because soon I'm going to ask you a very important question. Everything you feel, expressing it to the other person or other people, out of your body, out of your mind, out of the spaces you've been holding it in all these years, and you know where those spaces are inside of you. You're releasing it right from your gut, your back, your head, your heart, wherever you've been holding it. And this is right. Accepting and expressing. This is the right thing to do, always has been, always will be. This is right. Beautiful.

Okay. Now when you're ready in the next minute, or now, whenever you're ready, here comes one of the most important questions, a healing question, a very powerful question that you need to go inside to answer, and watch what a difference this makes in how you feel forever and ever about the unfinished business and about these people. Here's the question: What do you want this person or these people to say back to you now? And with your non-dominant hand and just allowing it to move across the paper, what do you want—after expressing all this, saying all this, letting go of all this, being real, being total, being 100 percent, now what do you want this other person or these other people to say back to you? A sentence, a word, more, less, I don't know. Go ahead and write it down. What do you want this person or these people to say back to you?

The Parent Trap

There's a special category of unfinished business that almost all of us need to deal with: Our relationship with our parents. I hate to pick on parents—I'm a father myself—but the truth is they usually had quite a bit to do with our issues. When it comes specifically to weight problems, our parents more than likely taught us our attitude toward food, modeled for us our eating habits, and are responsible for much of the emotional weight we carry around within us.

You see, our feelings toward our parents are often a mixture of love and resentment. Our mother and/or father were, after all, our primary source of love, support, and security; but they were also (in their role of socializer or disciplinarian) our primary source of punishment, criticism, fear, guilt, and restriction. Our relationship with them is thus almost always filled with positives and negatives, with gratitude and with regret, with caring and with anger, with sweet memories and with bitter. This is why we have such a sense of conflict about our parents, and why we so often repress our feelings about them.

So if you want to finish with all your old business, get it done with and then move on in life, you simply have to settle some things with your parents. One way to do this is to have your parents (or parent) on stage with you in the previous trance scenario. Talk to them honestly about how they hurt you while you were growing up: "This went on for years and years and years, from the time I was one until I was nineteen, and the only reason it stopped then was because I moved out!" Really let go. Say it all. Don't hold back.

And if it gets to be too much, breathe and take a break as the Second Watcher in the last row. But no more holding back, thinking things like, "a good son or daughter wouldn't feel this way," or "a nice person wouldn't have reacted the way I've reacted"—because that's what caused all the stress, and all the emotional weight, in the first place. You hold it in, hold it in with all these judgments about yourself. So my advice is, say it all. Let it go.

The beautiful thing about this technique, too, is that you don't ever actually have to confront your parents. You say it, let it go, and finish with it for yourself, in your self-hypnosis work, and then you're done with it. You resolve it on your own and then when you're with your parents, if they're still alive and still a part of your life, you have this perspective on them which is wonderful.

Expressing in self-hypnosis works wonders, but you can also let go and have done with things in slightly more realistic ways. Try this exercise.

Pick up the phone and unplug it.

Call your father or mother, or whoever raised you. Make it a three-way call if need be.

Let them know about the two biggest mistakes they made in raising you. Let them know how much they screwed you up. Ask for an explanation of their actions or inactions. Be direct, "I feel. . . ." Be honest. Be tough. Say everything you feel, and get it all out. Once and for all.

Now, after expressing everything you feel to your parents, ask them the life-changing question: What would you like to say back to me?

Listen carefully.

Now, tell your parents the two things you most appreciated about how they raised you. Be direct. Be honest. Be kind.

Tell them goodbye.

Plug the phone back in and call the number to get the time and date.

Let go . . . let go . . . let go.

Put Your Past Behind You

Another way of thinking about repressed thoughts and feelings is to understand that your past has somehow jumped off the time line of your life and gotten way too involved with your present and your future. It's wise to consult your past every so often, to ask its advice on current matters, and to use its experience to help guide you forward. But you mustn't allow your past to take the lead in your life, making you relive the same pattern of experience—eating to find love and comfort, for example—

over and over again. In a sense, you need to put the past behind you, where it belongs.

The following trance scenario can help you put your past in its place.

> *Focus on your breathing and I hope that during the days and nights ahead you take at least one or two or three breaths a day where you simply focus on the rise and fall of each breath. You unconditionally accept your breathing as it is and you pause a little bit at the turning points. And at your own pace I want you to think about a weight-loss issue that's been concerning you, that's been stressful or difficult for you, anything at all, something from childhood, something from your teenage years, something from your early adult life, and I want you to picture that issue and I want you to see what's happening in that situation.*
>
> *So you're seeing yourself or maybe you're getting a feeling for yourself, maybe you're seeing other people, getting a feeling for them. All I want you to do is get an image of the problem that's been troubling or concerning you, and I want you to notice if it's black and white or in color. I want you to notice if it's big or small. And I want you to see if there are any details that you can see or feel about this weight issue and notice where it is, probably in front of you. Maybe it's right in front of you, right in the center. Maybe it's a little to the right. Maybe it's a little to the left. Maybe it's a little bit up. Maybe it's a little bit low. It really doesn't matter. Just see the issue, the situation, yourself, the problem, the concern, and just kind of get a sense of where it is in front of you, almost like you could reach out and touch it right in front of you, real big or to the right or left or color or black and white.*
>
> *And once you see or feel where it is, with your breathing and your imagery allow it to move a little bit to the*

side, still in front of you, a little right or a little left, but still in front of you. Once that's happened, same issue, same situation, you're not trying to change a thing, let it move a little farther left or a little farther right but still in front of you so you have to look to the side or feel where it is, in front of you to the right or to the left. Once it's there, let it move beside you, either right or left so it's no longer in front but it's to the side and you can see it. You can sense it. You can feel it.

And once it's to the side of you, either side, let it move about a foot or two feet behind you, so still to the side, maybe two or three feet to the side. I don't know. And now a little bit behind you, say one or two feet. And once it's there, just one or two feet behind you, maybe two or three feet beside you, let it move a little farther back, maybe three or four or five feet behind you, still beside you, two, three, four, five feet beside, and now behind you three, four, five feet behind you. Once it's there, let it move maybe six or seven or eight or nine or ten feet behind you, still two or three or four or five feet beside you, but six, seven, eight, nine, ten feet behind you.

Same issue, same situation and let it get farther back, maybe twenty feet, maybe fifty feet, maybe more. But now it's way behind you. Same situation, same conflict, same concern, way behind you and off to the side. And once it's there, just keep it there because the past is always behind you. You're always in the present. And now look and just kind of see what's in front of you. It's probably looking very clear and very open, so maybe focus on a goal or a success that you want to have in your life. It's very different looking out at the future when things are clear, as opposed to when you have to look through the past to the future.

So now the past is way behind you. That issue, that conflict is way back there. You're in the present. You can breathe and feel yourself in the present and now you

*can see your goal or where you're headed very clearly, a lot
of openness out in front of you. Now, memorize this experience. Always keeping the past behind you and the present
headed towards the future, so when things come up in the
past you know where they belong. If you want to work on
issues like you know how to now, you can bring them up
from way back behind you in the past, bring them in front
of you. Do the committee work, finish with the unfinished
business. Do whatever work you need to do. And then when
you're done, that's right, put it back where it belongs way
behind you.*

*Now as you memorize this, stay with your breath work
because this can help you remember, that's right, because
your breathing is the bridge between your innermost self
and your outermost self. So take a couple of moments. Take
a minute. Take whatever time you want. When you're 100
percent sure you have this memorized, that's right, use your
breathing as the bridge. Stretch your arms or legs. Feel well
rested and refreshed at your own pace. That's right.*

Give Your Shame a Voice

Because it's such a painfully ingrown emotion, shame is one
of the most difficult barriers to overcome in anyone's life. Most
of us carry a bag of it around with us nearly everywhere we go.
Overweight people carry an especially big bag. The only way to
let go of shame is to stop living with it choked inside and give it
a voice of its own, as in these exercises:

1. Pull the telephone plug out. Check to make sure that it's
   definitely unplugged.

   Now dial 911 or 1-800-FBI, CIA, the police.
   Tell them all the bad, shameful things you've ever done.

Tell them about everything you think they might be even remotely interested in, from the time you were a little child to what you did this morning.

Laugh . . . shake . . . scream . . . cry, but tell them. Everything. Secrets, skeletons in the closet, disgraces, evil thoughts, humiliations. Everything.

In a week call them again, and report that you feel much better now.

Let go . . . let go . . . let go.

2. Make a list of all the shameful things you've ever done. Write small.

Make a list of all the kind things you've ever done. Write big.

Write a description of yourself based solely on your shameful deeds.

Write a description of yourself based solely on your kind deeds.

Imagine these two people meet. Write a script of the dialogue they might have. Imagine what the shameful person and the kind person would say to each other.

Enjoy the kindness you could offer the shamed person.

Let the two people embrace.

Let go . . . let go . . . let go.

Sexual Healing

Our sexuality is one of the most powerful drives within us, and sadly one of the major sources of shame and repression in our lives. If your shame is all mixed up with your sexual feelings or experiences, as it is for most of us, stop hiding or hating these emotional memories and let them go. The following exercises can help get you started:

1. Write a letter to a person you regret having sex with. Start it, "Dear _____,"

   Tell them what you remember about the experience. Write down your feelings, thoughts, and all the physical details you can remember.

   Tell them how the experience affected you. What it meant to you. Let it all out in this letter. Breathe deeply while writing.

   When you've finished the letter, take it outside. If you have a private mailbox, put the letter in it. If not, just pretend to do so.

   Leave the letter in the box for seventy-seven seconds.

   Take it out and read it slowly.

   Burn it.

   Let go . . . let go . . . let go.

2. Take a walk to a large body of water, the ocean, a vast lake, a broad river. Or just imagine it. Observe, listen, and breathe into the moment.

   Imagine you're on a voyage upon the water.

   Imagine adventure, love, lust, love, lust, adventure.

   Make the voyage last a long time. Observe, listen, and breathe into the moment.

   Remember how easy it was to take this voyage. Agree to take another each time you're near a body of water.

   Let go . . . let go . . . let go.

Express Your Stress

Stress is a killer, particularly for overweight people who are already putting extra strain on their heart. But just in general, most doctors agree that 75 percent of their patients' ailments are stress related. Nor is there much question that stress is the number one cause of weight problems (also of smoking, drinking, and many other chronic health problems). And what causes such killer stress? The research clearly suggests that the normal stresses and strains of daily life become dangerous when people repress their feelings about their problems and difficulties. Think about that for a moment. It's not the problems themselves, but people's repression of their feelings that elevates stress.

What this means is that the dangerous stress in your life comes from a war you're having with your own feelings; it's the inner conflict you're having as your feelings fight against being strangled and buried alive. You're fighting yourself, and you experience this conflict as stress, as muscle tension—your muscles are literally tensed for the struggle.

Now, since expression is the opposite of repression, I want to show you how you can effectively express the stress and tension out of your body.

One of the greatest relaxation techniques I know of was taught to me by Milton Erickson. He used this trance technique—what he called "Entrance–Exit"—on his own crippling pain, and I've used it in my own self-hypnosis ever since.

So make yourself as comfortable as possible, focus on your inhale and exhale. You might think of your breathing now as an entrance, that's the inhale, and as an exit, that's the exhale—entrance . . . exit. Beautiful, stay with it, get into a little routine . . .

> *What I want you to do now is focus on an area of your body where you feel some tension, or stress, or worry, or concern. Go ahead, actually focus on the difficulty, or stress, or worry, or concern. As you inhale, hold your stress or tension as tight as you can, exaggerate it, and then with your exhale let it go. Even say these words to yourself on the exhale, "let go." You can say them out loud or to yourself, it's up to you.*

Another thing you can do is focus on your body, from your toes to the top of your head, and squeeze and feel the tension in your whole body. Exaggerate the tension in your feet. Squeeze your hands, make a fist. Close your eyes real tight. Close your mouth real tight. Lift your shoulders up. Hold the tension just as long as you can, your whole body tense, tense, tense. And then let go and really relax, everything open, everything loose, kind of like a Raggedy Ann or Andy doll. Good, we're going to do this again. Bring in the tension. Squeeze everything, your hands, your eyes, your feet, your legs, your belly, squeeze it, hold the tension there. Lift your shoulders up toward the top of your head. When you're ready, when you can't hold it any longer, exhale and let go. What a difference. Entrance–Exit. One more time, squeeze your body, everything, get as tense as you can, shoulders up, fist clenched, feet, belly, jaws, everything. Hold it as long as possible, a little bit longer than you have the last few times, and now let go.

What you're learning to do is what I want you to continue doing with your breathing, with tension, with worry, even with discomfort: I want you to exaggerate it, let it enter, hold it as long as you can, be aware of it as long as you can, and then let go and release it.

That's a present from Dr. Erickson to me, to you.

Whenever you do this trance, you're taking time to take care of yourself in some fundamental ways. Instead of denying and holding in your stress, you're actually expressing it loud and clear, and then you're letting go of it. What you're going to find is that, because you've been practicing the Entrance–Exit technique, you'll instinctively start to relax any time you feel stressed, worried, tense, or in some discomfort. You'll just let things enter, let things exit, stress and relaxation, inhales and exhales, entrance and exit.

A nice variation of this technique can help you let go of stress in specific areas of your body. If you've used Entrance–Exit or Jacobson's progressive relaxation and found some stubborn tension in a knee, in your stomach, in your neck, anywhere, you can flow right into this scenario . . .

> *Scanning your whole body, from your toes to the top of your head, be aware of tension and stress in certain places. Wherever the tension is, place one of your hands directly on that spot. That's right, actually lift your hand up and put it right on the spot where the tension is, and say these two words aloud, but softly, and directly to the area: "Please relax, please relax, please relax." Continue moving to other parts of your body where there's any tension left at all, lay your hand right there on the area, and say these two words: "Please relax, please relax, please relax." So you're talking directly to the area with your hand there and you continue going through your whole body, placing your hand right on the spot and communicating directly with this area with these two words: "Please relax, please relax, please relax."*

You'll find that, after just a few weeks of practice, you'll only need to put your hand in the area and it will automatically know to respond in the same way. Then after a few months of practice, you'll only have to think about the area and say those two words to yourself, and the area will let go and begin to relax.

There are times, however, when you just have to let go physically. You have to get the muscles really involved. You have to sweat it out. Try this exercise:

> *Find an outdoor location where you can get physical— perhaps a garden to dig in, a playground to kick a ball in, a wood pile to chop, a stream to throw rocks into, a park to run in, or the like.*

Remember what feeling is blocked and feel that feeling as intensely as you can. Say the words, "let go" while expressing the feeling. Or if you can find a secluded place, scream or grunt the words out as you . . .

Dig out the feeling.

Kick out the feeling.

Chop out the feeling.

Throw away the feeling.

Run off the feeling.

Let go . . . let go . . . let go.

Artistic Expression

Art is a medium of expression all too few of us take the time to explore or play around with. But it's one of the best ways to let go of feelings and memories because it's a direct channel to your creative, unconscious mind.

Now, you don't have to go to art school to make art; be self-taught, and self-expressive:

1. Go to an art store and buy some drawing paper and a box of crayons, colored pencils, or some brushes and paints.

   Find a location to do your drawing or painting.
   Remember the worst experience of your life. Remember how you felt.
   Draw or paint the experience. Create the shapes and the figures, the scenery and the dimensions of the negatives.
   Use the colors you think best represent the negative feelings you had then.

When you've finished, look at your picture. Talk to it. Yell at it. Cry at it.
Let go . . . let go . . . let go.

2. Choose another sheet of paper.

Think of the best experience you've ever had. Remember how you felt.
Draw or paint the experience. Create the shapes and the figures, the scenery and the dimensions of the positives.
Use the colors you think best represent the positive feelings you had then.
When you've finished, look at your picture. Talk to it. Sing to it. Laugh with it. Dance around it.
Let go . . . let go . . . let go.

Music is an even more powerful way to get your feelings out. If you play an instrument, learn some pieces that express your deepest emotions. Or just play free-form with notes and chords that capture the feelings inside you. Playing drums is great for expressing all sorts of feelings because they're easy to fool around with and they really get your body involved.

If you don't play an instrument, use recorded music to get in touch with your emotions. For instance, if you're sad, play some great old blues songs and let yourself get deeply into the music. Breathe with the singer or in rhythm with the song and let go when the number is over. Or, even better, turn an emotional piece of music up louder than usual and dance to it. Slow or fast, it doesn't really matter. Traditional steps or free-form, it doesn't really matter. Just let your body say all that needs to be said.

Writing can also help you give your emotions a voice. Keep a journal and write in it daily about what you feel. Jot down images, lines of poetry, character sketches, bits of dialogue that come to you, dreams, passages from books you're reading, anything you want. For example, here's a fragment of two-hundred-year-old poetry that speaks to the whole "modern" issue of repression and expression. It's from a poem called *A Poison Tree* by William Blake:

> I was angry with my friend:
> I told my wrath, my wrath did end.
> I was angry with my foe:
> I told it not, my wrath did grow.

Simple words, simple rhymes, but expressing an eternal truth.

The Big Red Hot-Air Balloon

You'll be looking on the positive side of things even more in the next chapter, as you learn about replacing food and eating with new and healthier solutions to your problems. But for now, I want to leave you with one of my very favorite trance techniques for letting go of your emotional weight: The Big Red Hot-Air Balloon.

Get comfortable in your chair, take several deep, cleansing breaths, and feel your hands or your feet getting heavy, your jaw relaxing . . .

> *Imagine this and let your imagination be as playful as you want. You're taking a walk outdoors in a beautiful grassy field. You can feel the sun shining and feel its warmth on your body, a slight cool breeze blowing by, the grasses bending just enough to be beautiful and graceful, and the birds floating and flying in the bright blue sky. And you notice there's a great big meadow off to the side, and in the middle of the meadow is a great big, red hot-air balloon and it grabs your curiosity. Like a little kid, you wonder about it.*

It's kind of unusual in the middle of a big meadow to see such a great big, red hot-air balloon. So because you're curious and maybe because you're surprised—I don't know, maybe you're more surprised than curious (it really doesn't matter)—you want to see it up close.

You walk down towards this great big, red hot-air balloon and as you get closer to it, you see it has a big basket under it, you know the kind you can go for a ride in. There's no one in the basket, so you look inside and see there's a container. You reach inside and pick up the container, and find it's empty. It's almost as if the container was all set up perfectly for you to load in all your unfinished business, any stress, any problems, any extra hassles that have been in your life. And you start filling the container with your negative thoughts, your guilt, stress, hassles, worries, just filling it and filling it, old stuff, new stuff, current stuff, past stuff, little stuff, big stuff, getting the stress out of your chest, the guilt out of your head, the worry out of your stomach. And as you're filling the container, you start feeling lighter and more comfortable. And the more stuff you put in, the better you feel, until the container is all full. And when it's all full, you start to feel really better and more comfortable and relieved and kind of happy about this amazing opportunity that you've discovered.

And then you notice there are sandbags holding the red hot-air balloon to the ground, tied to the basket by big, thick pieces of rope. But you see a knife nearby and with it you to start to cut the sandbags loose. So you cut the first sandbag loose and when you do, you feel like you're letting go, cutting the cords to the stress, and the worry, and the hassles. And this is a great feeling. And then you go to the next piece of rope and the next sandbag and you cut that one and you feel even better, like you're really letting go, feeling really free and comfortable. And you go to the next one, cut that one loose and now this great big, red hot-air balloon is starting to lift a little bit off the ground and that feels even better. And you go all the way around and you cut all the sandbags loose and you really feel like you're letting go once and for all of all that unfinished stuff you put in the container.

And when you get to the last rope, and cut the last sandbag loose, naturally all your concerns start lifting up and away from you as this great big, red hot-air balloon starts lifting into the sky. And as it leaves the ground, there's a great, comfortable feeling of letting go and releasing. And as it floats higher in the sky, you feel even better. You may even feel like waving goodbye, it just feels so good to see all that stress, and worry, and guilt, and difficulty floating away. And the higher it gets, the better you feel. The higher it soars, the lighter and freer you feel. And pretty soon that great big, red hot-air balloon is just a red circle in the blue sky and it keeps getting higher and higher and farther and farther away and you feel lighter and freer and more relaxed, happy. Pretty soon, it's just a little red dot in the great big, blue sky. It's a great feeling. It's a Second Watcher kind of feeling, free, relaxed, happy knowing that you know how to do this for yourself anytime, any place. You can do this every day. You can do this whenever you need to. It's a way of taking care of yourself and a way that's just a wonderful opportunity, whether you do it for a couple of minutes or a couple of moments, for ten minutes or two minutes. It really doesn't matter.

And so now you know how to let go. Now you know how to release. Now you know how to feel better anytime, any place with this great big, red hot-air balloon. And whenever you're ready, whenever you want to, with your non-dominant hand, just draw a picture of this hot-air balloon. Write the words of how you feel after you let go of all that stress that went up and up and up and farther and *farther away. How do you feel? That's right. When do you want to do this again? A fun way to let go and take care of yourself. You've got to love it. This is what it's all about. That's right. That's right.*

So say goodbye to all the weighty issues, thoughts, feelings, memories, experiences—all of what you've been holding on to and carrying around inside for so long. Let it all go, and start to live again. Expression is life. Expression is life-giving, it's energizing, it's inspiring, and it's the pathway to new resolutions and new perspectives. Live an expressive life, and you live a life of creativity and joy. Learn how to express your *self*, and you'll be living in a natural way, you'll be listening to your intuition, listening to your body, listening to your heart, listening to your intelligence, and trusting yourself to go where your spontaneity takes you.

CHAPTER 12

Phase Four: Resolution

Now that you've come to the last phase of the Keep It Off Weight-loss program, let's look again at the idea we began with: Overeating is not your problem in life; it's your solution to the problems in your life. When your personal life feels empty, or when you're deeply dissatisfied with yourself or your relationships, or when you've stuffed yourself with repressed emotions that only leave you feeling hollower and hungrier, you try to solve the problem with food. You eat and overeat to fulfill yourself, to satisfy yourself, to comfort yourself, to make yourself feel better.

This is the solution you've come up with, and it works, at least for the moment. But the sad reality is that it doesn't work in the long run. In fact, it does terrible harm. You eat to feel better, and you overeat because it does feel good, and so you get overweight—and then your problems multiply. You hate your weight, and your body, and yourself (and others) even more than before, and you also invite a host of medical problems, including diabetes, heart disease, cancer, back pain, the list goes on and on.

Soon your doctor tells you to diet and exercise, or perhaps in disgust you find a book that says to eat more protein, or more carbs, or not to mix the two—or some new twist—and maybe you lose some weight. But then you lose your commitment, your focus, and you start eating again, and you gain back all the weight, and more. What's wrong with this picture?

The truth is that the same old solutions are always going to keep coming up with the same old results. And this is because the underlying personal, emotional problems are still with you, still controlling you, still trying to get your attention, and they're ready to trigger the cycle all over again.

If you want to get finally free of your weight problem, to kick the old habits for good, you need to find new solutions, new answers, new discoveries, new perspectives, new understandings. You need to "re-solve" your problems in a way that will work for you, and that will keep on working.

What you need is a breath of fresh "**AAER.**"

You've already read in this book how to become **A**ware of what's going on inside yourself and how to **A**ccept yourself as you are—these are the two key door openers to weight loss and weight management. You've also read how to **E**xpress your feelings, thoughts, and memories in order to close with the unfinished business and the old conflicts that have been controlling your life. So far, so good. Now this chapter will show you how to use self-hypnosis to find your own new **R**esolutions for a positive, healthy future.

You know, self-hypnosis does one thing wonderfully well. It allows you to access and to remove all the emotional and psychological barriers that society, family, and you, yourself, have erected in your life, barriers that have prevented you from creating your own better solutions to your problems. Everyone has problems, issues, and challenges in life, but no one is born with self-criticism, bad habits, negative conditioning, self-doubts, and self-limits. You're given these things, or you adopt them, as you grow up, and they become huge rocks in the road to realizing your potential for positive personal growth. Self-hypnosis gives you the skills you need to do the inner work that can remove these blocks—undo what's been done to you—and get you back on the road to health and happiness.

Make no mistake, this inner work is the crucial thing in losing weight and keeping it off. Weight Watchers works and Jenny Craig works and Overeaters Anonymous works, and the whole exercise and nutrition thing works just fine—*if*, that is, you've done the inner work. But if you haven't done the inner work, if you haven't learned about awareness, acceptance, expression, and resolution, none of the plans or programs work. None of them help. Or they help maybe 5 percent of their clients, if they're lucky.

By learning self-hypnosis, however, and by practicing the trance techniques and inner exercises in this book, you're going to become more self-aware, more self-accepting, more open and expressive, more intuitive. You're going to learn to be kind to yourself, compassionate, and to take responsibility for your own self-care. You're going to feel really centered, really alive, more relaxed, more confident, and more in harmony with life. You're going to get in a beautiful flow that makes life a daily celebration.

Oh, and by the way, you'll be losing weight and keeping it off as a side effect, a byproduct of your new and healthier way of life.

What Do I Do Well?

All too often people approach trying to solve their problems with sneaking thoughts of failure. They want to do well and find answers, but the memory of their faults and past failings casts a shadow on their confidence and subtly, insidiously undermines their efforts.

So the first thing to learn about resolving your weight-loss problem—or any other problem—is how to trust yourself and build on what you do well.

Go ahead, if you haven't already, focus on your breathing, and maybe go to the Second Watcher on the mountaintop and observe yourself as you relax. Sometimes it's helpful to ask yourself this question, or some question like this: How relaxed can I feel right now? Repeat that question to yourself (and not out loud) ten or twenty times until you really feel a change and a positive click, a positive yes. How relaxed can I feel right now? Take all the time you need to make yourself feel as comfortable and relaxed as possible . . .

> *I want you to focus, using your third eye perhaps, on one thing you do well. Maybe it's being a good friend, maybe it's playing tennis, maybe it's being a parent, maybe it's working with people or working on your computer, maybe it's gardening or cooking or being open to new ideas. Anything from A to Z, from your childhood or your adulthood. Whether it seems more playful than important, or more serious than fun, it really doesn't matter. I just want you to focus on one thing you do well, because if you can do one thing well, you can do anything well. That's right.*
>
> *Now, whatever you're thinking about right now, whatever you're picturing in your mind, whatever you're feeling in your body, focus on this thing you do well and be as specific as possible with yourself about the details of how you learned to do it. Of course, you had to be a novice to begin with, everybody starts that way. But how did you go from knowing next to nothing about it to becoming good at it? What was the process? That's what I'm asking you. What did you have to do to get good at this one thing? What were the steps? What was the formula? Did you read a book? Did you need a coach? Did you write about it? Did you talk to other people about it? How much time and energy did you put into it? How long did it take? Did you have any breakthroughs along the way? How exactly did you learn to do this one thing well?*
>
> *Remember details that maybe you've forgotten, or that you haven't thought about in a long time. Get into it, be*

that age, live in that home, be at that job, and remember and actually re-experience, relive how you went from knowing very little or nothing to doing a thing so well. Use all your senses. See it. Feel it. Hear the conversations. Smell the place. Remember the taste you had for learning this new thing and becoming really proficient, really competent at it. You may be surprised about some things. I don't know. But take these minutes to remember the steps. That's right. Use the Second Watcher perspective, step way, way, way, way back and see how you did it. See what had to happen. See what you had to do. Learn and remember just as much as possible about your formula because I'm going to ask you an important question in just a minute but not yet. Good.

Okay, once you have enough information, enough details, and you can feel it, you're not just thinking about it but you can feel it, start to apply this process, this formula, to your losing weight and keeping it off, to your self-care and relaxation. What do you need to do? What are the steps? What's the process? Knowing you, knowing what works, knowing what's already worked for you, utilizing a past success and applying it to your present goal, your formula, your method. You already have this inside of you. You've been doing it for a long time and now you're applying what already works for you to your present goal, your number one priority. Do you need to do more reading? Do you need to do more practicing? Do you need to do it every day? Do you need to talk to other people? Whatever you did to become good at that one thing, apply all of that formula to your losing weight and keeping it off, to self-care and relaxation.

Enjoy the process. Enjoy the journey. You're discovering that if you can do one thing well, you can do anything well. Take a couple of more minutes and focus on what it took for you to do that one thing well and apply it to your number one priority, same formula, same steps, same process, *apply it to what's really important to you and what you're working on now. Stay with it. Stay with it. Be playful about it. Be serious about it. Have fun with it. Be focused. Remember the whole premise here. That's right. If you can do one thing well, you can do anything well.*

You've been opening up a lot of new doors, developing a lot of new resources, finding new answers inside yourself. Take another few minutes with this before you finish. You already know that often, just before you finish, something really important clicks inside. And from a deep place, you get something that you're always going to remember. So now, at your own pace, when you feel really good about what you've done here, start to finish up. And as you've probably already guessed, go back to your breathing. Go back to focusing on the rise and fall of each breath. That's right. Accept your breathing as it is and pause with awareness at the turning points. That's right. Finishing up with this, because your breathing is the bridge between your innermost self and your outermost self. That's right.

Positive Self-Talk

Learning from your past successes is important, but perhaps even more important is learning to support and encourage yourself with positive self-talk.

One of the significant discoveries in psychology in recent years has been our understanding of the role our own casual self-talk plays in the shaping of our lives and our bodies. For example, how can you expect much success with weight loss and weight (self) management when you're continually telling yourself things like, "I'm going nowhere in my life, I just can't do this, Every time I try to change I fail, I just don't like me, Why should I try if it's not going to work anyway, I'm no good, I'll always be fat, Just this once won't hurt, I can't help myself, I don't know what's wrong with me, I've tried but I just can't."

These are the kinds of messages we've heard about ourselves from others, messages we've heard so often that they've come to define our own self-image and to direct our daily lives.

How much better you could be doing if you were saying to yourself things like, "I'm making progress with my self-care, I can handle this, I'm getting free of my triggers, I'm willing to try, I'm good at this, Just this once I won't, I feel more accepting and loving towards myself all the time, I feel especially good about my new skills, I'll keep trying self-hypnosis and I'll get it."

Unfortunately, very few of us have been taught how to have this sort of positive attitude about ourselves. On the contrary, from childhood we've been programmed by our parents and teachers (well-intentioned, no doubt) to be negative about ourselves, to humble ourselves, to limit ourselves, fearing that, if given our freedom, we might become too arrogant and egotistical, too assertive and outspoken and disobedient.

Eventually we grow up and take charge of our lives, but the old programs continue to control our self-talk, our self-care, and thus our weight and body image. And so we reach adulthood overweight and gaining more weight as the years go by. Then we're faced with a dilemma: Do we settle for the body we were programmed to have, or do we try to change somehow, go back to self-care school now when we're on our own, and find our real, authentic body?

If we leave our self-care to chance, as we had to do as children, we can be certain that we'll fare no better in the future. Our bodies will be the mirror of our negative self-talk. Unless we do something for ourselves now, we're destined to live out our lives mismanaged and unsatisfied.

The decision is ours. We can manage ourselves with negative words that discourage us and lead to weight gain, or with positive words that give us confidence and encourage weight loss.

Self-hypnosis is the best way I know of to reprogram self-talk, which makes it perhaps the most powerful tool available for building a new positive attitude about your weight and your body. To change your attitude, or inner atmosphere, I want you to repeat any eight of the following sentences, or any ones like them, in your trance sessions at least once a day:

"I accept my body and I am glad that it is working as well as it is."

"I'm glad to be alive and I've decided to take the best care of my health I can."

"Today is a really good day; I'll have other good days, but today is special."

"Today I choose to relax about my relationships and eat healthy all day."

"I can do it—just watch me."

"I take responsibility for my self; only I determine how I look, how I feel, the choices I make, and the decision to eat intelligently."

"I only eat foods that are good for me."

"I enjoy eating right."

"Eating a meal or a snack, I taste every bite, eat slowly, and relax in the present."

"I consistently eat like a person who weighs _____ pounds. (*This should be the goal weight that you've decided on.*)

"I know that how I look, what I weigh, and how I feel are 100 percent my responsibility, and each day, each night and each moment I do everything I can to create the real me."

"I've already decided and am 100 percent committed to taking care of myself—and that includes how I look and what I weigh."

"I know the best way to lose weight and keep it off is to believe in myself, feel free in choices, and see my self the way I really want to be."

"I know my weight depends totally on my perspective, and I see myself as becoming lighter, healthier, and happier, everyday."

"Each day, before I get out of bed in the morning, I relax and become aware of my new self. I set my goals, I see myself achieving them, and I love them."

"I'm ready, willing and able to do what it takes to feel and look the healthy way I want to. It may be difficult but I'm worth it."

"The more I listen to my Second Watcher, the more I recognize the true, authentic me (inside and out)."

Give this exercise some time for a few weeks, and you'll soon find yourself integrating positive self-talk into your life each day, all day.

The Committee Meeting, Part 4

You can also use the Committee Meeting strategy to manage all the various voices or committee members in your head—positive or negative. As I've explained in previous chapters, these committee members might be your many thoughts and feelings on the weight issue, or they might be you at different times in your life, or they might be various sides of yourself that all need to be heard before you make any firm commitment about losing weight and keeping it off. You might seat many committee members, or few; it doesn't really matter. As long as they're all acknowledged, accepted, and listened to, you'll be open to new learning, new experiences, new perspectives, and you'll be able to come up with a resolution or "committee report" that takes all opinions and attitudes into account.

Here's a tightly focused committee meeting that's particularly effective for resolving weight issues. First, take a piece of paper and at the top write down these four words: Body, Heart, Mind, and Intuition. Next, jot down your goal: Losing Weight and Keeping It Off.

Now get as comfortable as you can. With paper and pencil available, focus on your breathing, on the rise and fall of each breath. Accept your breathing as it is and notice that your breathing has a rhythm, with the inhale probably different from the exhale. Your breathing might be fast or slow, belly or throat, small or big. No matter. Whenever you accept your breathing as it is, you get a glimpse of yourself, of your true being, and what it feels like to accept yourself as you are. Put your awareness on the turning points, and see if you can pause a moment at the turning points. When your inhale turns into an exhale, and when your exhale turns into an inhale, just pause a moment. You're focusing on the rise and fall of each breath, just like waves at the beach. They roll in, they roll out. It doesn't matter if they're big or small, deep or shallow, colorful or not. Accept your breathing as it is and then pause at the turning points, just for a moment, just at the moment of quiet, the moment of peace. Okay, good . . .

> *Now with your pencil in your non-dominant hand, I want you to get in touch with how your body feels about your weight issue. Be aware of your physical body from the bottom of your feet all the way to the top of your head. How does your body feel? Is there any tension? Any tightness? Feel any stress anywhere? You know, my body feels kind of tense, I feel it in my stomach or kind of in the back of my*

neck. You're doodling, scribbling, drawing pictures, writ-ing words. If your body could talk, if your body had a voice of its own about your weight, what would your body say? I feel . . . here's where my tension is . . . here's where I hurt . . . this is where my discomfort is.

Give your body a voice and express whatever your body is feeling about your goals. And it may be things you've been noticing for a long time, or maybe brand new stuff that you're just getting in touch with now. Let your body express itself. No more repressing in your body. No more pushing things down in your body. This is your body talk. This is your body language. Take a couple of minutes and let your body talk. Let your body express itself. This is your opportunity to say yes to your body. Whatever you feel, whatever you want to say, put onto the paper. That's right. Take another minute.

And when you're ready, use your breathing as the bridge to transition from your body to your heart, focus on the rise and fall of each breath and pause a little bit at the turning points. Ask yourself, how does your heart feel about the issue? It's not literally your heart. It's your heart as a metaphor for how you feel. What are your feel-ings about losing weight? You might notice your feelings right across your chest, right in between your armpits. A lot of times people say they feel really closed and tight right there when they're stressed, and a lot of people say they feel warm and open there when they're relaxed. What are the feelings? What are your emotions?

If your heart had a voice and your heart could talk, what would it say about this issue? What would it say about this goal? Accept what you feel. Express what you feel. Give your heart a chance to talk. You've heard the expression heartfelt feelings. No more pushing down. No more holding in. No more holding back, everything your heart feels about this issue. That's right. Finally, you have an opportunity, right here, right now, to give your heart a voice, to express your feelings about your weight, and take a couple of minutes. Let go, let go, let go. Be all heart. Be all heart for yourself and give your heart a voice. That's right. Be all heart with yourself.

Focus again on your breath work, at your own pace. Focus on the rise and fall of each breath. Just like the waves at the beach, they roll in and roll out. Accept your breathing as it is. Pause a little at the turning points. And use your breathing as the bridge to go to your mind, your thinking, your intelligence, your ideas, your theories. What does your mind say about losing weight? Your mind is very different from your body and your heart. Your mind is your thinking and maybe you have a lot of thoughts, a lot of views, a lot of opinions. Maybe you've always had a lot of thoughts. What are you thinking about? What are your ideas about your weight? What are your concerns about it? What's your mind been thinking? What kind of worries, doubts, reluctance, ambivalence? Any thoughts at all. Give your intelligence a voice. What does it say?

And just allow your mind to express, to communicate, to be heard, from your head to your hand to the paper. What does your mind say? Maybe what you thought it would say, maybe more, maybe less. That's right. What does your mind say? Take a couple more minutes. Maybe it seems like you've been stuck in your head on this issue. Maybe you feel like you've been overthinking it or perhaps not thinking about it enough. I don't know. It really doesn't matter. Just allow your mind, your ideas, your thoughts, your intelligence to have a chance to have a voice, to express itself about losing weight and keeping it off.

And at your own pace, your breathing as the bridge, focusing on the rise and fall of each breath, accepting your breathing as it is and pausing a little bit at the turning points, ask yourself, what does your intuition say about los-

*ing weight and keeping it off? And just allow your intui-
tion to bubble up. First with your non-dominant hand and
then with your dominant hand, what does your intuition
say about this issue? You've heard from your body. You've
heard from your heart. You've heard from your mind. Now
what does your intuition say? Most people think of their intuition as in their gut, kind of a gut feeling. But really it's
your true, authentic self, some might call it your soul. It's
your voice, your deepest inner voice. It's your observer, or your
Second Watcher, that curious, friendly, compassionate part of
you that's open to new solutions. It's your voice of resolution.*

*And so, from this Second Watcher perspective, last row,
mountaintop, big picture, comfortably detached, loving,
accepting, what bubbles up? What comes to you as the best
resolution to this issue? Just take your time. It may be exactly what you expected. It may be completely different. It
may be very simple. It may be quite complex. From the
Second Watcher, with your non-dominant hand, what's the
best resolution to the issue?*

*And just wait and wait and be patient and wonder
what your intuition is going to come up with. Anything
at all. Perhaps you've already written it down or you're
about to or you're in the midst of writing it now. What's
the best resolution to this issue from the last row? Remember, this is the truest you. This Second Watcher, this intuition, this inner voice is closer than maybe you've ever been
to your true, authentic self. What's the best resolution?*

*Feel free to give your intuition a voice first with your
non-dominant hand and then with your dominant hand.
Listen to your intuition. Express it onto the paper. Feel
how freeing it is to let your intuition go. And trust that
when you're 100 percent about giving your body a voice,
and 100 percent about giving your heart a voice, and
100 percent about giving your mind a voice, your intuition will come shining through with 100 percent. And this*

is what's meant by being whole, by being your true self, by honoring yourself, accepting yourself, mind, body, heart, and soul. You've heard that before. Listen and be guided by your own mind, body, heart, and soul. That's right.

So take a couple of minutes. Use your breathing as the bridge. And at your own pace, feeling well rested, refreshed, maybe like you've been napping. When you're ready, stretch your arms, your legs, count from one to ten, and feel wide-awake.

One last word about committee meetings. If you do your committee work for all your big issues, and hold meetings on a regular basis, one day you'll be done with them. After a while the process will become second nature, and you'll do the awareness, accepting, expressing, and resolving without even thinking about it. It's like when you were a child learning how to read. First you studied the alphabet, you practiced the letters, you memorized them, you started to sound out words, *ka*, *da*, *ba*. But pretty soon you just knew how to read, and you didn't have to go back and sound out every syllable; the process simply became a natural part of your consciousness. That's exactly what happens with the Committee Meeting technique. At first it takes some time and effort, but soon it becomes internalized and you're doing it unconsciously.

Conflict Resolution

Naturally, smaller conflicts occur in everyday life—am I going to have the salad or the cheeseburger for lunch?—and you don't always need to call a full committee meeting to resolve them. When little things come up, you can stay focused on your goal of being healthy, happy, losing weight, and keeping it off, if you've developed some basic skills in conflict resolution.

Here's a simple and fun idea to try.

Whenever you're dealing with a conflict, whenever you're having difficulty deciding something, it helps to write down a quick list of the pro's and con's. So whatever the issue is— something at work, or something about food, or something about your body—you're going to make a list of the pro's and the con's. And you're going to focus on how you feel about both sides. It doesn't matter whether it has to do with exercise, or with meals, or with relationships. You're just going to make a list of all the pro's and con's. See which list is longer. That's a good start.

Now the fun part. After you've made your list, imagine a split-screen TV, with part of you talking about the pros on one side, and part of you talking about the cons on the other side. Or if you watch those political debate shows, like *Crossfire*, imagine yourself speaking for the resolution, and then speaking against it. Most important, while each part of you is making its points, let yourself come together out of the TV and sit watching the show from the sofa or a chair. From this observer perspective, you'll come up with your best resolution.

Script Your Future

You've probably observed that awareness, acceptance, and expression all focus primarily on the past and the present, from your childhood to yourself as you are now. Resolution, on the other hand, tends to look to the future. You base your resolutions on past and present factors, of course, but you make them with your eye on the future, on your goals, your intentions, your hopes and dreams, on the way you want to be.

A good way to understand this is to extend your work on "Unfinished Business" from Chapter 11. Let's set the scene: Your Second Watcher has left the last row of the theater and has walked up on stage to confront some troubling figures and memories from the past—to let go and say everything needed to heal some old wounds. Let yourself breathe comfortably into trance, focusing on the turning points between each inhale and exhale, and pausing for a moment to feel the peace. Maybe look down from the mountaintop and see the big picture, feeling friendly, caring, and compassionate toward yourself. Eyes growing heavy, if they aren't already . . .

So you've been accepting all your own feelings today and you've been expressing all your own feelings today. And now you're in the process of resolving all your own feelings today. This is going to make a big difference in a lot of ways, and from now on you're going to feel, better, different, healthier, healed, whole, free. There are lots of ways to describe it. And after you've expressed what you want to this person or these people, and after you've listened carefully to what they had to say back to you, use your breathing as the bridge and, at your own pace, go down the steps on the side of the stage, if you haven't already, and all the way back up the aisle to the last row.

And when you get there, from the Second Watcher, last row perspective, having watched everything that just happened up on the stage, you letting go, expressing everything you feel, after you got it all out and heard what that person or those people said back to you, now from the Second Watcher, from the last row, what is the best resolution? What do you see? What do you feel? What do you know? What do you like about what happened just now on the stage, while you were finishing with the unfinished business? And for the past few minutes, while you've been doing all this, from the Second Watcher, how do you feel? What are your feelings and impressions about everything that just happened, about everything you just did? What do you feel? What do you like? What difference do you already notice? And how do you want things to go from now on?

In other words, after doing all this accepting and let-

ting go, write the script of how you want things to go. You're the playwright, you're the director, and the producer too. So imagine the script changes you want. Make the rewrites. Change the plot, change the dialogue. From this moment forward, I want. . . . That's right. How do you want things to go from now on? That's right.

Explore What's Possible

Let's not forget that the real focus of self-hypnosis is on the present, on becoming happy and healthy in your life right now. As I've said many times, the past is always behind you, the future is always in front of you, and you're forever in the present. But just as dealing with your past can help free you from it, so looking to the future can help you focus on your target and achieve your goals. So let's take some time now to think, maybe even meditate, about what your life is going to be like in the future.

What's actually possible for you now that wasn't possible before you started this book, before you made the commitment to lose weight and keep it off? What's possible just in terms of how much better you feel about yourself now? What's possible in terms of your personal relationships with others? You have options. You're thinking about your decisions and the consequences. What's possible in terms of your health and your appearance? What's possible in terms of work, and love, and personal fulfillment, family and friends and so on? And with your weight, your food problem, what's possible now?

This is a perfect time to take out your journal and write down and describe what you expect of your life. How do you want it to go? What changes do you want to experience? Write down everything you can about your desires, your intentions, your passions, and your commitments. Be specific. Make plans that are reachable, doable, and imagine your sense of accomplishment as you complete them. And definitely make them fun. How do you want to look and feel, physically, mentally, emotionally, or even spiritually? What's it going to be like to be completely free of the weight and food issues, self-esteem issues, and relationship issues?

Focus with an open mind, and an open heart, and a total commitment to developing your potential. Write down the new ways that you'll take care of *you*. Write about the new things that you want to add to your life, to your routines, any new activities, any new feelings, any new behaviors, new opportunities, even new perspectives. Be open to describing everything in your writing about what you want one month from now, three months from now, then six months, one year from now, even five years from now. What about ten years from now, or in the far, far future? You see, you're making plans to make your life freer and happier. You're writing about how you'll deal with problems. You're writing about being calm in rough times. You're writing about resting fully when you go to bed at night. You're writing about how great it feels to make a transformation from your very core. You can write about a renewed love for life, about flexibility, about being open to exploring. Maybe you're even writing poetry or drawing. You can write about pacing yourself, self-acceptance, self-love, health, enjoyment, and freedom.

Now write in your journal about your freedom from the old, unwanted habits of being overweight, about your commitment, about your wisdom, about your ability to see things with different eyes, and your ever-evolving nature. Write about being proactive instead of reactive. Write about being flexible rather than rigid. Write about living each day fully and breathing fully. And about relaxing a little bit everyday. And about integrating your new feelings, your self-respect, and your self-acceptance.

The point to remember is that you have the power to write your own life script or life story. If you're open to new ideas and options, and if you nourish your intentions to be healthy, happy, to take care of yourself and your body, you can be the author of your own future.

Two Crystal Balls

Another powerful way of describing your future is by visualizing or picturing how you want to be. Here's a trance technique to help you see into tomorrow. As always, take several deep, cleansing breaths, and relax with the techniques you've found most effective . . .

Imagine two crystal balls. Gaze into the first and see your life and your weight problems in the future, if you stay the way you are now. See yourself, your body, your eating habits, your clothes size, your social life, your private time, and everything else that will happen (or won't happen) if you keep doing the same old things you've been doing for years to try to lose weight. Maybe you see yourself losing the weight and gaining it all back (and maybe even more). Maybe you see yourself trying different exercise programs and not sticking with them. Maybe you see yourself just eating in the same old familiar ways and not doing anything except gaining more and more weight. This is the crystal ball that shows your life in the near future, and the far, far future, if you do nothing to change it.

Next, look into the second crystal ball. This one shows your life and weight in the future, if you do what you can to change. Which means: You learn self-hypnosis, and practice with your breath work and the Second Watcher. You learn to relax and develop new self-care skills. You deal with your issues from the past and resolve them. You develop a friendly, caring, and compassionate relationship with yourself, your body, your emotions, your intelligence, and your intuition. Maybe you see yourself happier and healthier and lighter than you've been in decades. Maybe you see yourself eating more slowly, making better choices, and nurturing yourself in all kinds of new ways. Maybe you see yourself being more physically active, eating more intelligently, losing weight and keeping it off. Maybe you see yourself in the clothes you want to wear, or in a new bathing suit. Maybe you picture the size you want to be, how much stamina you want to have, how strong you want to feel, what your weight is, how your hair looks, even things like your posture. This is the crystal ball that shows your life in the near future, and in the far, far future, if you learn how to change.

When you finish your trance, you might begin to understand just how much you can trust yourself. You know what to do. You've always known. You just didn't know how to do it before. That's what you're learning in this book. You can look into the crystal balls as often as you wish. You're learning how to see things with different eyes.

Embrace Your Future

By imagining how you want to be and behave in the future, you're actually creating a relationship between your present self and your future self. The following trance allows you to develop that relationship with love and respect.

Get into your open, receptive mood with your breathing, maybe with some stretching, maybe reminding yourself the past is miles behind you, the future is miles in front of you. If you feel any tension put your hand on the place and say, "please relax, please relax . . ."

You're going on a journey, following a path that's in front of you, because the future is always in front of you, and you're seeing the beautiful trees, noticing that even though you can't see the roots of the trees you know they're down there, and that's a really solid feeling. And you're noticing the clouds up in the sky and just watching the clouds go by one at a time, just as you've learned to watch your own thoughts go by like clouds in the sky, here one comes, there it goes. And as you're watching the clouds, you can put a thought into each cloud and just watch them come and watch them go. They're always temporary. That's one thing you know for sure.

And you notice way up the path, sitting at the base of a magnificent old tree, there's a person, looks like a grown person, can't really make it out from here, but you're curious, open, you have a sense of adventure which you've been developing more and more on these journeys. And as you get closer and closer to that tree, it looks as if the person sitting at the base of the tree is an older person and somebody that looks kind of familiar. And as you get closer and closer, you realize this person is a future you, an older version of yourself. And you walk right up and reach out, and the future you rises and reaches out, and you hold each other, you embrace each other. An incredible moment, a great feeling of closeness. And maybe you hold each other in a way that neither of you has felt in a long, long time, an embrace filled with love, and care, and compassion, that's right, really understood, really accepted.

And now a conversation can happen. Whatever you want to say to your future self, any questions you want to ask, that's fine. And of course, your future self is compassionate, and friendly, and open, and listening. And then whatever your future self wants to say to you, advice, encouragement, important changes you can make, challenges you'll face, you're open, and you listen. That's right. And

*now the conversation flows back and forth about relation-
ships, since you know relationships are the most important
thing about self-respect, and self-respect is the most important thing of all. That's right. You allow the dialogue, the
conversation to flow, allow yourself to be pleasantly surprised by your openness and your receptiveness to each other.*

*And only after you feel satisfied with the dialogue,
then you move yourself up to the Second Watcher perspective, all the way up to the mountaintop and watch. That's
right. Just watch. And then whenever you feel satisfied
and have some new ideas, you begin the journey back down
to where you started, seeing things with different eyes,
more clearly, learning things, open to new learning. That's
right. Really noticing where you're going to give your attention from now on, and feeling like you've just given
yourself a beautiful gift that you can bring along into the
future.*

Squaw Peak

To end this chapter on new solutions, on seeing with new
eyes, I want to share a magical coming-of-age story told to me
by Dr. Milton Erickson.

*There's a place in Arizona called Squaw Peak. It's quite a
big peak, and just a couple of hundred years ago an Indian
tribe lived at the bottom, and a family of rattlesnakes lived
way up at the top. In the tribe at the bottom of Squaw
Peak there was a youngster who really wanted to be a
grown-up, an elder, to be one of the adults. And so this
young Indian would always ask, day after day, week after
week, month after month, can I be an adult, can I be a
grown-up, can I be an elder, can I be one of you? And of
course just everyday things went on and on and on.*

At the top of Squaw Peak there was a young rattle-snake who really wanted to be accepted as one of the adult rattlesnakes and would always ask the adults, when can I be one of you, when can I be an adult, when can I be grown-up? And of course the everyday things went on and on and on. That's just how things went.

And then one fateful day, the adult Indians at the bot-tom of Squaw Peak went to this young Indian and said, to-day is the day you can become an adult. All you have to do is climb to the top of Squaw Peak, and when you get there look out and find us a new place to live where there's sun, and shade, and water. And the young Indian could hardly wait and started climbing, started to climb up Squaw Peak.

On the same fateful day, the adult rattlesnakes went to the young rattlesnake and said, today is the day, all you have to do to be an adult is go to the bottom of Squaw Peak, and when you get there look around and find us a new home where there's sun, and shade, and water. And the young rattlesnake started going right away.

About half way up and half way down, the young In-dian and the young rattlesnake came face to face, eye to eye, staring at each other, moving around each other cau-tiously. And each of them realized that they could fight, and one may die, one may live, both may die, who knows? They stood there staring at each other for what felt like an eternity. And after a long while, the young Indian started going back down Squaw Peak much slower than he walked up. The young rattlesnake started slithering back up Squaw Peak much slower than he had come down.

Finally back down at the bottom of Squaw Peak, the young Indian told the adult Indians what happened in a sad, dejected, unhappy voice. And all of the adult Indians said together to this young Indian, welcome, you are now one of us. Self-respect is the most important thing.

And at the top of Squaw Peak when the rattlesnake finally got there, he told the adult rattlesnakes what had happened, and he was sad, dejected, and unhappy. But the adult rattlesnakes all at the same time said to the young rattlesnake, welcome, you are now one of us. Self-respect is the most important thing.

What's the point of the story? It's hard to say, but maybe it means that there are positive alternatives in every situation, if you have the courage to take them. Maybe it means that your real goal in life is not social acceptance but integrity and self-respect. Or maybe it means that personal growth and evolution happens from the inside out.

You can enjoy more and more of your life, free from the emotional and physical weight that has imprisoned you for so long, but it all begins with how you feel about yourself. Be respectful, be supportive, be caring, be concerned, be compassionate, be understanding with yourself. Listen to your commitments. Learn to take care of yourself the way you would take care of a person you really loved and really cared about. Feed yourself that way and you'll grow into the future you've dreamed for yourself.

CHAPTER 13

Challenges and Successes

I just want to take this time to say from my heart how really happy I am for you, the reader. You've devoted all this time and energy to yourself. You know you're worth it and you've proven it by staying with this book and reading through all the self-hypnosis techniques I've suggested. And hopefully you've begun to practice some of them and make them part of you—part of your heart, part of your mind, part of your soul, part of your body. It takes a lot of courage, determination, and a positive regard for yourself to make this commitment to a whole new way of life, and to take up inner work like this. You can feel really proud of yourself now.

But I would be less than honest with you if I didn't say that you're going to face some challenges ahead as you shed your pounds and your programming. There's always an integration period, or learning curve, in a process this powerful, and you're going to have moments of doubt and relapse. For some people this learning period can be days. With other people it can be weeks. And with others it can be months. Fortunately, you know from your self-hypnosis work that difficult times, like your thoughts and feelings, are always temporary.

Challenges

With every success, every time you breathe through a craving, or let a temptation go by (just like a cloud in the sky), you can enjoy your new freedom. Still, at other times it's not going to be easy. At times you're going to get cravings, and a part of you will want to revert back to your old eating habits. At times the people and the situations that trigger your eating will be so powerful that you'll want to forget your commitment and go back to what's been familiar. And at times emotions may build up in what feels like overwhelming proportions, and overeating may seem easier than giving them a voice in a committee meeting.

Sometimes you may feel that you aren't getting the support you need from a loved one, or a co-worker, or a friend. And sometimes, you may feel you're finished with your food and relationship issues, only to be tested by loved ones, or friends, or co-workers who still have issues themselves, who are still stuck in committee. Some days you may just have a bad day and you'll say to yourself, oh I just want some chocolate today for comfort—like a call from a sweet old boy or girlfriend. And the list of situations you might encounter could go on and on.

In addition, and let's be honest, sometimes you're going to slip up and overeat. It's normal, and it's going to happen. Expect to be tempted, it's part of the movie, it's part of the process, it's a totally natural thing. Expect that your cravings are going to come up, and that you may even give into them some of the time. Expect people and situations to trigger you, and expect it to be just too much some of the time. Expect that there will be times when you just want to go back to that old familiar way of eating and not taking care of yourself—that old routine that you relied on to help you through hard times. Expect that there will be a part of you that needs that crutch again.

Your greatest challenge may be to stay committed to being your true self, and not beat yourself up or make yourself feel worthless if you slip up a few times. We all have a tendency to get way too upset with ourselves when we slip and fall, or when we even think about it. And it really doesn't make any sense. Remember when you learned to ride a bicycle as a child. Didn't you fall down a few times before you really found your balance and mastered the ride?

So be gentle with yourself. Be flexible with yourself. No matter what, there's no need to be judgmental or critical of occasional relapses. It's all part of letting go. Give yourself some room to be human and to make progress. You know the old saying, two steps forward, one step back. You can let go of trying to be perfect about your weight and your eating. But you can enjoy being perfectly okay!

Successes

Relax and know that you've come an extraordinary distance already. Please take a moment to really acknowledge your progress. Think of the courage it took just to buy this book and to begin the whole journey in the first place. And now you've learned how to get in touch with significant emotional memories from your past. You know more about how to live in and enjoy the present. And you've discovered the secrets of how to resolve your problems and take care of yourself in the future.

You now have the possibility to achieve something extraordinary in your life. I hope that you'll take from this book a new confidence, a feeling of exhilaration, an empowering strength that will help you stay on course and reach your final goals—to lose weight and keep it off.

As you've been reading this book, you might have been

wondering, can this program work for me? Frankly, that will depend on your commitment, on your determination to do what it takes from now on to remain light, relaxed, and in balance. There's no magic bullet or wonder supplement here. There are no miracles with self-hypnosis.

But I can promise you that the principles of self-hypnosis and the specific techniques and exercises I've detailed in this book have helped thousands of real people with their weight loss and weight management problems. Here are just a few success stories, both case histories from my files, and statements from a number of my recent patients.

> **Pam:** "I really have enjoyed the classes with Dr. Alman and learning self-hypnosis. I've found that the most important thing about taking these classes has been that it's made me realize how much my mind is the most important part of weight loss. Everything else I've done, all the programs I've been involved in, everything I've done, it's always been that I've concentrated on my body or on outside focuses in attempting to lose and control the weight loss. Now I've come to realize that it is my mind that determines what happens with my body and with the self that is going to be whatever weight I want to be. I started out in the program at 227 pounds, a year and a half ago, January of 2002. And in January of 2003, I weighed 140 pounds and I've been maintaining that, and I like that weight, and I find that by using the steps that Dr. Alman has suggested, I'm able to maintain that weight. I like the program and I enjoy working with the people involved in it."

> "**My** appetite is a lot smaller than it used to be and it's much more satisfying."

> "**From** the smaller portion I serve myself, I get all the pleasure, nourishment, and satisfaction that I need."

"**I can** take as long as I need to eat, and I'm more assertive with others, and I like it."

Dave: "Hi. I just want to say thanks to Brian for an unbelievable class. Brian has changed my whole attitude and the way I think about handling stress and about handling my eating disorder problems. And he's helped me. Whenever I think about going to the refrigerator to start breathing right, I do the little things, the techniques that he has taught us, and it's really helped me keep my weight. And it's helped me in all kinds of different situations that I've been in where I'm able to use his techniques to communicate, to be able to think through a process, to clear my mind. I told my daughter about several of the techniques that we were using and she is using them now in her classroom. Thank you."

The Case of Julie

At thirty-five, Julie hated to look at herself in the mirror. It seemed as though she'd been on a diet continuously since her first pregnancy twelve years ago. Then when her doctor urged her to find a way to control her overeating, Julie got pretty angry. "That's easy for you to say," she snapped. "You're not a waitress who's around food all day."

The doctor knew Julie had worked hard to support herself and her two children after her divorce three years before. He could sympathize that waiting tables all day sapped her strength and motivation to exercise in the evening. "All I want to do is go to sleep so that I can get up each morning and start my routine all over again," Julie told him.

When the doctor suggested self-hypnosis to help her change her eating habits, Julie didn't take him seriously. But a few days later, after overhearing two customers make a cruel joke about her size, she decided it was time to try a new approach to losing weight. She called her doctor and made an appointment to begin instruction in self-hypnosis.

In the early sessions, Julie discovered how much hurt and resentment she felt toward the women who had made the joke, toward thin people, toward her ex-husband, and even toward her parents who had divorced when she was ten. Julie had repressed all these feelings for years, not wanting her kids to feel the confusion and rejection she'd experienced as a child.

But now she began to write about her hurt, anger, and resentment in a personal journal each night. As Julie accepted her right to have these feelings, she gradually learned to let go of them by giving them a voice of their own.

Next, she decided to explore the possibility that she might be overeating to satisfy her emotional cravings rather than physical hungers. By keeping a record of what foods she ate each day and how she was feeling when she ate them, Julie realized that she consumed more when she was lonely or bored. And she was lonely and bored so often! She wondered if she might be using her weight as an excuse to avoid meeting people.

As Julie learned more about herself through self-hypnosis, her enthusiasm for life began to return. She remembered books she'd enjoyed as a child and read them again to her own children. One night, while listening to some old 1950s rock-and-roll records, she began to dance to the music in her living room and was surprised to recall her natural sense of rhythm. She was soon dancing every night, thrilled to have found a form of exercise she enjoyed.

Encouraged by these successes, Julie used post-hypnotic suggestions to resist excessive eating during the day. Through her trance work, she learned to alter the way she looked at food. The results were dramatic.

Julie lost sixty-five pounds in nine months. When an acquaintance at work asked her for her secret, Julie loaned her a few record albums and promised to teach her some dance steps. It wasn't long before the other waitresses joined in. They decided to throw a 1950s dance party at the restaurant, and the evening was such a hit that everyone decided to make it an annual event.

Julie made more and more friends and found she was less bored and lonely. Although her hours at work hadn't changed and she was still around food all day, the excess weight stayed off. Two years later Julie was attending a dance class three nights a week, enjoying her life, and liking the way she looked.

"I enjoy exercising more now than ever before. I'm living my commitment. I believe in myself and my attitude is I'm proud of myself."

Peter: "I've lost 85 pounds since I've been in the Kaiser program. I started in 1988 and I maintained for about nine years, and then up again forty pounds. And so I went through the program again, and I lost forty, the forty that I had gained. At first I was a little reluctant about going into the self-hypnosis training with Dr. Alman, and I am thankful that I did because I've found out I'm probably a stress eater. And the program has taught me how to deal with stress and I think I'll have a better chance at success of maintaining."

"**Every day,** instead of gaining weight, I'm gaining self-esteem."

The Case of Steven

At the age of forty-five, Steven was proud to be able to buy his two sons the things his own father had not been able to afford. As a sales manager for a prominent manufacturing company, Steven was required to travel frequently, and he spent many of his evenings wining and dining important clients. But he knew he would receive a big promotion if he could increase his company's sales by just 3 percent. Sacrificing a few years of his personal life now seemed a small price to pay for financial security later.

Steven had always been slightly overweight, and he had tried various diets for the past seven years without much success. Steven's doctor said the problem was a lack of control over his eating habits, but Steven believed it was a lack of exercise. Since his hectic schedule made regular exercise difficult, he exhausted himself with grueling physical workouts on the few weekends he was home. He hated these sessions, knowing they were only guilty attempts to shed extra pounds put on by stressful drinking and overeating at business lunches and dinners.

During one particularly strenuous workout, Steven hurt his back and was confined to bed for two weeks. Panicked by the thought of the company's sales suffering during his absence, he spent long hours trying to conduct business on the telephone in his bedroom. When he wasn't barking orders at his sales force or badgering clients, Steven ate junk food and stared gloomily at the TV.

When he was at last able to return to work with the help of pain medication, Steven found he couldn't put in the long hours he had been able to handle before his injury. And as his work and worry increased, he lashed out at everyone around him. His family and friends accused him of being impossible to get along with. He knew in his heart they were right. Steven hated the person he was becoming, but it seemed he couldn't control his pain, his temper, or his lifestyle. To make matters worse, he found he was gaining weight even faster than before. Finally, in desperation, he sought help through self-hypnosis.

Within one month, Steven had learned the techniques of self-hypnosis well enough to gain some relief from his back pain and to encourage mild exercise. He began to look forward to taking daily walks regardless of where his travel schedule took him. Away from the pressures of his office or the loneliness of his hotel room, Steven was able to get in touch with his true wants and desires by practicing self-hypnosis.

He realized he was lonely and began to accept his need to be a father and a husband. He resolved to rework his tough travel schedule and save the weekends for family outings and camping trips. He decided he deserved to enjoy the life he had right now, not what it *could* be sometime in the future.

To alter his eating habits, Steven cut back on the heavy restaurant meals in the evenings, and, as an experiment, he invited one client for breakfast at a simple, family-style restaurant where cocktails were not served. Steven was pleased at how much was accomplished in this bright, cheery atmosphere, and he planned similar breakfasts with other clients. He soon discovered that many people enjoyed meeting in the mornings rather than at the end of a long exhausting, frustrating day.

After three months of self-hypnosis, Steven had lost fifteen pounds. His decision to spend weekends at home allowed him to enjoy his family life more than before, and his life improved in other areas as well.

Since his walks made him feel so refreshed and revitalized, he gave himself post-hypnotic suggestions to recall those feelings whenever his nerves became jangled during the business day. As he gained more self-acceptance, he became a more effective manager. Members of his sales force remarked on the change in him and he found it easier to communicate with them.

Within six months the company sales increased by 5 percent, and Steven was promoted to Vice President of Sales. He lost ten more pounds and reached his own comfortable, healthy weight, and, more importantly, he finally felt free to manage his own life.

Nancy: "Self-hypnosis with Dr. Alman have really been a big help to me in the last number of weeks. I have a lot of chronic pain, and also a weight problem. And what's happened is by being able to deal with the pain, and get a great deal of relief using his methods I've been taught, I am also able to control my eating, and I've been continuing to lose weight on this program, not just maintain. And between losing the weight and by feeling better with the lessening, a great deal lessening of my pain, I am doing more exercising and getting around. Life is just a whole lot better. And I know that I'm going to get to the goals that I've set for myself as far as weight, and it's really made a major difference in my life both with weight loss and my weight-loss goals, and my freedom from pain."

Ruth: "I've lost 118 pounds due to Dr. Alman's self-hypnosis program, and I wanted to come to get more self-hypnosis training to be able to maintain my weight when I do reach my goal. I think that the two most important things that I've learned are acceptance and awareness, being aware of who I am, how I got to where I was, and where I'm going, what I'm going to do with it. Acceptance is the key to being able to make those changes and be able to put the techniques that we used in Dr. Alman's self-hypnosis program to work for me."

Bob: "I've lost and gained over 100 pounds three times in my adult life, tried different programs of weight loss and the emphasis usually was on just diet and exercise without much talk about the mental aspect of it. The tools that I've learned as a result of Dr. Alman's self-hypnosis work have enabled me to have something that's readily available and that they're easy to learn, and I can use them throughout the day. And I think it's been a very good addition to my weight-loss plan."

"As I'm losing weight, I'm finding it easier than I thought to maintain my new image. My new eating habits are easier to keep because they are my habits, ones that I've created myself."

Barbara: "I've just completed Dr. Brian Alman's program, Self-Hypnosis for Weight Loss, and it was a very positive and useful experience for me. Dr. Alman teaches in a very clear, supportive way and he offers many, many tools and techniques to support a positive lifestyle. I learned techniques to help me explore ways that I sabotage my own best interest in terms of weight management, weight control. I learned tools for uncovering triggers that lead to my over-eating. I also learned many methods to support my positive habits and behaviors, not only in weight management and weight control, but also in all areas of my life where I want to rid myself of addictions and unproductive behaviors. I now have a much fuller toolbox, many tools and techniques that I can use right now, but also for the rest of my life when I want to work on change, and just in terms of supporting my own growth and healing as I move on in life. So I would highly recommend the program to everyone. Not only those who are concerned about their weight and weight issues, but for everyone because we all have issues of self-esteem, habits that we aren't happy with, behaviors we want to change, and Dr. Alman's program not only supports all these things, but really helped me to move toward a greater sense of self-empowerment."

Through self-hypnosis all of these people, and many, many more like them, have learned to redirect their internal resources to achieve their goals. Because they decided to deal with their inner, emotional weight—the pounds and programming they'd been carrying around for years, and allowing to control their lives—they were successful in shedding their outer, physical weight and in keeping it off. In self-hypnosis, they found the only weight-loss program they would ever need.

Now as you finish this book, it's time to trust yourself. You know what to do. Take care of yourself, you're worth it. Right now state your commitment to losing weight, keeping it off, and achieving the freedom in life you've dreamed about. You deserve the best life you can imagine.

CHAPTER 14

Quick Program Guide

It's often said that every journey begins with the first step. So what's the first step in the Keep It Off Weight-loss Program? What do you do the first day? the first week? And where do you go from there? In Chapters 9–12 I presented the **AAER** roadmap, and offered a number of remarkably effective exercises and trance ideas as vehicles for change. But now I'd like to get practical and summarize just exactly how you proceed on your journey to better health, self-care, and permanent weight loss.

The following guide will take you safely and efficiently through the basic Keep It Off program. As always, you're encouraged to experiment with your own personal pace and preferences. But for the first few weeks, try to give your exercises and practice sessions around thirty minutes a day. As you become more experienced with self-hypnosis and more familiar with the program, you'll probably be able to cut your trance sessions to, say, ten minutes a day, five days a week. And soon you'll only need to practice five minutes a day, three times a week, to get the results you want.

Let's begin.

Week One: Getting Started

Work through Part I of this book one step at a time:

Session 1. In a notebook or journal you've dedicated to this program, please write down your **Weight-Loss Goals** (pp. 16–20). Be clear and detailed about what you want to accomplish. Make your goals specific and attainable. If your final objective requires a major change for you, set up specific intermediate goals (p. 20).

Session 2. Write out several different kinds of hypnotic **Suggestions** (pp. 22–26) for your goal. Design your suggestions using your own personal symbols and metaphors. Draw from your past experiences, dreams, work, play, and memories to develop effective personalized suggestion language. Use **Imagery** (pp. 23–26) and **Symbols** (pp. 23–27) to add power to your suggestions. "See, feel, hear, smell, and taste" your suggestions and the results you're seeking. Refer to Chapter 3 for lots of examples.

Session 3. Examine your **Motivation** (pp. 28–31) toward your goals and write down any underlying blocks to your success. Some of your deep-seated reasons for *not* wanting to lose weight might not be completely clear at this time. But even if you feel only hints of mental or emotional obstacles, write them down and say as much as you can about them in your notebook.

Session 4. Begin learning how to do **Healthy Breathing** (pp. 32–33) and **Progressive Relaxation** (pp. 35–38), either active or passive. Mastering these two methods is vital to achieving the kind of success you want in the Keep It Off program. Breathe and relax each day for ten minutes and you'll acquire skills that will benefit you the rest of your life.

Session 5. Practice some basic trance induction techniques in Chapter 5, such as **Eye Fixation** (pp. 40–42), **The Candle Flame** (pp. 44–45), and **The Stairway** (p. 45), to get familiar and comfortable with the feeling of entering a self-hypnotic trance. Take some time to explore a few trance scenarios from Chapter 6, such as **Breathing Colors** (pp. 55–56), **Fly Away** (pp. 60–62), or **The Mountain Climber** (p. 65). Pay special attention to **The Second Watcher** trance (pp. 63–64), because it introduces one of the most essential benefits of self-hypnosis—the ability to see your body, your weight, your emotions, your life with different eyes. Also, start to familiarize yourself with **The Committee Meeting** trance (pp. 66–68) because you'll be returning to it throughout the program.

Session 6. Give some thought to creating **Posthypnotic Suggestions and Cues** (pp. 71–73) to extend the influence of your self-hypnosis beyond your trance sessions and into your everyday life. For example, picking up a fork at mealtime might signal you to take a breath and slow down your eating.

Session 7. Slowly read through the sample **Trance Script** (pp. 77–84) in Chapter 8 several times and get a feel for how it's put together: entrance, development, and ending.

Week Two: Awareness

Continue practicing your breathing and relaxing each day, integrating them when possible into the following steps:

Session 1. Take the **Oceana Quiz for Emotional Weight** (p. 91) and begin exploring the emotional issues that are at the root of your overeating. In an age-regression trance (p. 96), **Explore the Starting Point:** How old were you when you first gained weight? Why *then*, do you think? Why not five years earlier or five years later? Just as importantly, what were your emotions around this time? In your notebook, please write down the age you were when you first gained weight, and write a few sentences explaining what feelings were troubling you at the time. Remember, nobody is born overweight. Weight gain does not come on gradually; it spikes up when emotional issues are stuffed inside.

Session 2. Start investigating your inner **Resistance** to losing weight. Work through the exercises on pp. 98–99 and write down what are, for you, the advantages of being overweight. Also, question yourself hard about your real **Motivation** for losing weight (p. 99). The honest answers might surprise you.

Session 3. Practice becoming aware of your **Feelings**. Pick a moment, any moment will do, and ask yourself, what am I feeling right now? Frustrated, bored, angry, hopeless, ashamed, or what? Now practice **Breathing Awareness** (p. 100) as a mirror to your inner feelings. In your notebook, please write down what you're feeling right now—frustrated, bored, angry, hopeless, ashamed, or what?—and note how you're breathing.

Session 4. Start observing your emotional **Eating Triggers** (pp. 101–102) and how they connect to your **Cravings** for food. In the midst of a craving, take out your notebook and write down what you're really hungry for. Also practice breathing through your craving (p. 100), a skill that you'll find useful in a thousand everyday situations. With greater awareness you can breathe through anything.

Session 5. In trance, hold a **Committee Meeting** (p. 103) to give voice to all the jumble of feelings involved in your craving for food. Also, learn about your **Programming Pause Buttons** (pp. 105–106), and practice **Humming** (p. 105) and **Gibberish** (p. 106) to interrupt your cravings, urges, and automatic responses.

Session 6. Become more aware of your food and how you eat. Learn the difference between **Tension Food** and **Relaxation Food** (pp. 107–109). Discover **The Joy of Eating** (pp. 109–110) and learn **The Fine Art of Eating** (pp. 110–111).

Session 7. Focus on your conscious and unconscious **Commitment** to lose weight. In the morning, please write down in your notebook your weight-loss **Priorities** for the day. Then, write down how much time you are going to give to each of your priorities that day. If possible, do this everyday! Also, engage your unconscious mind as you get up in the morning and at night before bed (pp. 112–113). And in a **last breath** trance (p. 113), help your commitment be absorbed into every cell in your body.

Week Three: Acceptance

Begin turning your new self-awareness into an active agent of change by accepting yourself, even loving yourself, just as you are:

Session 1. Practice observing and accepting your breathing exactly as you find it. If you're not breathing fully, you cannot be living fully. When your breathing is relaxed, everything else moves into alignment. Do the **Breath of Life** trance (pp. 116–117) at least three times this week, and also in your notebook write down or draw a picture that reminds you to be aware of your inhale and exhale . . . and to accept your breathing however it is.

Session 2. The next big step is to begin learning to accept *all* your feelings about yourself and your weight. Do the **Committee Meeting, Part 2** trance (p. 118) and be sure to write down and save the list of feelings you develop in this trance session. Next read the story of **Barbara** (pp. 122–123) and begin considering how powerfully the need for love figures into overeating and weight gain. Also study the **Yin Yang** meditation (pp. 123–125) to help you understand how "good" and "bad" feelings balance and depend on each other.

Session 3. Lightening up on your self-criticism is important if you're going to accept yourself as you are. Read and absorb the **Not Perfect, but Perfectly Okay** meditation (p. 125), and get in touch with the lighter side of your mistakes and failings with the **Blooper** trance (pp. 126–127).

Session 4. Do the **Hug Your Child** (pp. 127–130) trance several times this week, to help yourself make peace with your past experiences and failings, and begin to take better care of yourself in the future. Breaking with your past also means **Deprogramming** your automatic eating habits, which is the subject of the meditation on pp. 130–131.

Session 5. Fundamental to any success with long–term weight-loss is accepting your body as it is. If you hate your body you'll never do what's healthy for it, but you can begin to develop a positive body image by doing the nude **Body Perspective** exercise (pp. 131–133) for one minute every morning and night this week. Also get a larger perspective on the natural right-ness of your body with the **Tree Roots** trance (pp. 133–135), and take a moment to appreciate the miracle that your body is by doing the **Thank Your Body** trance (p. 135).

Session 6. You can deepen your attitude of acceptance by learning to observe the objects and the people around you for what they are, without judgment or criticism. Do the **Gaining Insight** trance (p. 136), and the **Accepting Others As They Are** age trance (pp. 138–140), to give you some ex-perience looking past the surface of things.

Session 7. Self-acceptance is the ultimate goal of this week's work, and the **Speak Your Name** trance (p. 140) will take you deep into your own identity. Once there, you'll understand that you don't need to please everyone else, or meet others' expectations. And by considering the One/Third Theory (p. 142) you'll realize that trying to please everyone else doesn't work anyway.

Week Four: Expression

Awareness and acceptance are like the inhale of a deep, satisfying breath; and now, with expression, you start to exhale and let go of your old habits.

Session 1. To get the juices flowing, do the mental and physical **Letting It Go** exercises (p. 145). Follow this with the **Committee Meeting, Part 3** trance (pp. 146–150) in which you scribble or doodle in your notebook whatever each of your committee members/emotions needs to say. No more holding in; let all your feelings have their say—from your heart to your head to your hand.

Session 2. Finishing with your **Unfinished Business** means expressing how you feel about the hurts and wounds you've received over the years, so that you can let go of your old coping devices and get on with life. Do the Second Watcher trance (pp. 151–154) and make sure you write down whatever you and the key people in your life—particularly your parents!—need to say to each other. Get it all off your chest. You might also want to try the exercise in **The Parent Trap** (pp. 154–156).

Session 3. If you've allowed your past to have too much power in your life, too much control over your present, devote a whole self-hypnosis session to the long **Put Your Past Behind You** trance (pp. 156–159).

Session 4. Most of us carry a burden of regret around with us and refuse to open up about it, and these repressed feelings and memories drive us to all sorts of excesses—including overeating—to help us feel better. Do the two **Shame** release exercises (pp. 159–160), and then go on to the two **Sexual Healing** exercises (pp. 160–161).

Session 5. Stress is essentially the pressure of bottled up emotions, so do the Entrance–Exit trance (pp. 162–164) to help release the tension you're carrying inside. Also try the please relax variation (p. 164), and do the physical sweat it out exercise (p. 165) at least once during the week.

Session 6. This might be hard for some of you, but make an effort to express yourself artistically this week. Do the drawing exercises (pp. 165–166), and get into playing or listening to some emotional music—even try dancing to it. At the very least, try writing some poetry or a story in your notebook. (See p. 166 for some ideas.)

Session 7. Let your work this week culminate in a full session with this compelling trance, **The Big Red Hot-Air Balloon** (pp. 167–170). Let your *self* soar with this image of healing, energizing emotional release.

Week Five: Resolution

Self-awareness, self-acceptance, and self-expression all lay the groundwork for resolution—the personal reorganization that means lasting change.

Session 1. To help you quiet your self-doubts, work through the **What Do I Do Well?** trance (pp. 173–176), and follow up with some writing in your notebook. Drawing on your trance work, write down the thing you do well. Now, write down what it took you to learn how to do this one thing well. Next, write down what you need to do to apply these same skills to losing weight and keeping it off. Finally, write down what you can do today to continue with your journey to lose weight and keep it off—using the skills that you already have inside of you.

Session 2. Start turning your outlook in a more positive direction by learning about the power of **Positive Self-Talk** (pp. 176–179). Also, in your notebook, make a list of what is right about you today. Make a list of what is right about losing weight and keeping it off. Also, make a list of the things you choose to do—today—to help yourself lose weight and keep it off. Finally, make a list of all the kinds of physical activities that you enjoy and check off the physical activities that you will do, or have already done, today. Keep adding to your lists and read them everyday.

Session 3. In an extended trance session, hold a Committee Meeting in which you consult your body, heart, and mind (pp. 180–184) to come up with your own very best ideas for losing weight and living more healthfully. For smaller, everyday issues, practice the **Conflict Resolution** techniques (outlined on p. 184).

Session 4. Resolution, as in a New Year's resolution, suggests making a commitment toward achieving a brighter future. To that end, do the **Script Your Future** trance (p. 185), which moves you past your unfinished business (pp. 151–154) into a future that you create for yourself. In your notebook, make a list of all the things you want for your future. Make a list of the things you can do today to help your future come true. Remember, anything you do today that is good for you will help you in the future. And anything you do today that is good for your future will help you today!

Session 5. Follow the suggestions in **Explore What's Possible** (pp. 187–189) and write in your notebook or journal about what you expect from your life from now on. What is your passion? What do you care the most about? What do you do that makes you feel powerful and positive? What is your purpose? Is it to develop your potential a much as possible? Is it to contribute your abilities to the world and make it a better place? List of all the things you're passionate about. List what you can do today to connect with your passion. List of all the things you can do over the next two years to connect with your passion.

Session 6. To get your imagination/unconscious more involved, picture what your future might look like in the **Two Crystal Balls** trance (pp. 184–190) and reinforce your intuition by listing in your notebook all the things that will not change and how your life will be in two years—if you keep doing the same old things. Then list of all the things that will change and how your life will be in two years—as a result of learning how to be aware, accepting, expressive, and open to new resolutions. Also, you began by getting in touch with your childhood (pp. 150–156), now **Embrace Your Future** in a touching trance (pp. 190–192).

Session 7. Perhaps the greatest gift that self-hypnosis can give you is the ability to see your self and your life with new eyes. Read the story **Squaw Peak** (pp. 192–194) and learn that self-respect is the most important thing. Make a list in your notebook of all the things that you can do today to enhance your self-respect. Break the day up into three parts: morning, afternoon, and evening. What you can do today to enhance your self-respect through being open to new choices, new ideas, new behaviors, and new possibilities?

Week Six: Daily Practice

To continue getting the kind of results you want with the Keep It Off Weight-Loss Program, you need only to be reminded of those key trance forms that you should work into a personal daily practice routine:

1. Healthy Breathing: pp. 32–33, p. 100, pp. 116–117
2. Relaxation: pp. 35–38, p. 164
3. The Second Watcher: pp. 63–64, p. 65, pp. 151–154, p. 185
4. The Committee Meeting: pp. 66–68, p. 103, p. 118, pp. 146–150

In a few more weeks, when these hypnotic experiences have become deeply ingrained in you, you'll find that you're affected by them almost unconsciously throughout the day, or whenever the occasion calls for relaxing, reframing, or resolving. At most you'll need to spend five minutes a day to lose the weight you want—and to keep it off.